WP 210

A Colour Atlas of
Diseases of the Vulva

CHAPMAN & HALL MEDICAL ATLAS SERIES

Chapman & Hall's new series of highly illustrated books covers a broad spectrum of topics in clinical medicine and surgery. Each title is unique in that it deals with a specific subject in an authoritative and comprehensive manner.

All titles in the series are up to date and feature substantial amounts of top quality illustrative material, combining colour and black and white photographs and often specially developed line artwork.

Slide Atlases are also available for some of the titles in the series.

1. **A Colour Atlas of Endovascular Surgery**
   R.A. White and G. H. White
   Also available:
   A Slide Atlas of Endovascular Surgery

2. **A Colour Atlas of Heart Disease**
   G.C. Sutton and K.M. Fox

3. **A Colour Atlas of Breast Histopathology**
   M. Trojani

4. **A Text and Atlas of Strabismus Surgery**
   R. Richards
   Also available:
   A Slide Atlas of Strabismus Surgery

5. **A Text and Atlas of Integrated Colposcopy**
   M.C. Anderson, J.A. Jordon, A.R. Morse and F. Sharp
   Also available:
   A Slide Atlas of Colposcopy

6. **A Text and Atlas of Liver Ultrasound**
   H. Bismuth, F. Kunstlinger and D. Castaing

7. **A Colour Atlas of Nuclear Cardiology**
   M.L. Goris and J. Bretille

8. **A Colour Atlas of Diseases of the Vulva**
   C.M. Ridley, J.D. Oriel and A.J. Robinson

9. **A Colour Atlas of Burn Injuries**
   J.A. Clarke

10. **A Colour Atlas of Medical Entomology**
    N.R.H. Burgess and G.O. Cowan

11. **A Text and Atlas of Arterial Imaging**
    D.M. Cavaye and R.A. White

12. **A Colour Atlas of Respiratory Infections**
    J.T. Macfarlane, R.G. Finch and R.E. Cotton

13. **A Text and Atlas of Paediatric Orofacial Medicine and Pathology**
    R.K. Hall

The amount of supporting text varies: where the illustrations are backed-up by large amounts of integrated text the volume has been called 'A text and atlas' to indicate that it can be used not only as a high quality colour reference source but also as a textbook.

In preparation

A Text and Atlas of Clinical Retinopathies
P.M. Dodson, E.E. Kritzinger and D.G. Beevers

A Colour Atlas of Retinovascular Disease
S.T.D. Roxburgh, W.M. Haining and E. Rosen

A Colour Atlas of Forensic Medicine
J.K. Mason and A. Usher

A Colour Atlas of Neonatal Pathology
D. de Sa

A Colour Atlas of Diseases of the Vulva

C.M. Ridley
formerly Consultant Dermatologist
Elizabeth Garrett Anderson and Whittington Hospitals
London

J.D. Oriel
formerly Consultant Physician in Genitourinary Medicine
University College Hospital
London

A.J. Robinson
Consultant Physician in Genitourinary Medicine
University College Hospital
London

CHAPMAN & HALL MEDICAL
London · New York · Tokyo · Melbourne · Madras

**Published by Chapman & Hall, 2–6 Boundary Row,
London SE1 8HN**

Chapman & Hall, 2–6 Boundary Row, London SE1 8HN, UK

Blackie Academic & Professional, Wester Cleddens Road,
Bishopbriggs, Glasgow G64 2NZ, UK

Van Nostrand Reinhold Inc., 115 5th Avenue, New York,
NY 10003, USA

Chapman & Hall Japan, Thomson Publishing Japan,
Hirakawacho Nemoto Building, 6F, 1-7-11 Hirakawa-cho,
Chiyoda-ku, Tokyo 102, Japan

Chapman & Hall Australia, Thomas Nelson Australia, 102
Dodds Street, South Melbourne, Victoria 3205, Australia

Chapman & Hall India, R. Seshadri, 32 Second Main Road,
CIT East, Madras 600 035, India

First edition 1992

© 1992 C.M. Ridley, J.D. Oriel, A.J. Robinson

Designed by Thin Blue Line, London
Typeset in Palatino by Keyset Composition, Colchester,
Essex
Printed in Hong Kong

ISBN 0 412 36520   0 442 31688 7 (USA)

A catalogue record for this book is available from the British
Library

Contents

Preface · vi

Acknowledgements · vii

Introductory Guide to Lesions · 1

1 General Principles · 5

2 Infections · 9

3 Non-infective, Non-neoplastic Conditions · 33

4 Tumour-like Lesions and Cysts, and Tumours · 63

5 Miscellaneous Conditions · 77

6 Childhood Lesions · 83

7 Child Sexual Abuse · 95

Appendix A · 101
  Classification of neoplastic and non-neoplastic conditions · 102

Appendix B · 103
  Classification of vulvodynia · 104

Further Reading · 105

Index · 107

Preface

This atlas is intended to be helpful to the clinician, whether in genito-urinary medicine, gynaecology or dermatology, who seeks guidance on vulval lesions. It cannot serve as a textbook on all aspects of aetiology, pathology and management but we hope that the text will supplement the pictures to the extent of providing some basic information.

The rare conditions, of varying aetiology, that present as ambiguous genitalia — which are not strictly speaking diseases of the vulva — are noted as an important differential diagnosis of labial adhesions, a much more common occurrence, but are not given detailed consideration. Clearly such a condition would call for a referral to a particularly interested paediatrician or gynaecologist.

Child sexual abuse is considered in some detail because its signs are variable and easily confused with vulval disease, e.g. lichen sclerosus. Rape, however, which would present essentially with non-specific signs of trauma, with or without infection, and would depend otherwise on forensic evidence for diagnosis, is not.

It was decided not to design the atlas in sections on 'red lesions' 'white lesions', etc. — an approach that is perhaps more reasonably (and easily) applied to wild flowers or to birds than to vulval conditions. Such terms to some extent devalue the essential need for exact morphological description of what is often a complex and dynamic situation. However, in recognition of the fact that it may sometimes be difficult for the inexperienced to begin without a signpost, a list on these lines has been compiled; it precedes the general text and illustrations.

Appendix A sets out the current classification of non-infective neoplastic and non-neoplastic vulval disease, as well as the scheme it superseded. The so far less well-categorized vulvodynia is annotated in Appendix B.

Finally, there is a list of suggested reading covering all aspects of vulval disease.

Acknowledgements

We are grateful to the many colleagues, too many to list individually, who have so generously allowed us to see some of their patients. We are also grateful to those listed below, who kindly provided us with some of the photographs.

Dr E. Allason-Jones, Mr B. Bhogal, Dr A.J. Boakes, Dr C.G.D. Brook, Prof. L. Collier, Dr F. Davidson, Dr M.J. Godley, Dr G. Kinghorn, Mr J. Lawson, Dr S. Lucas, Mr A. MacLean, Dr D. Maybe, Mr J. Monaghan, Dr R. Ruiz-Maldonado, Mr J. Shepherd, Mr P. Walker, Dr A. Warin, Dr J. Watkeys, Dr P. Wiesniewski, Dr J. Wynne.

We are also indebted to the publishers Churchill Livingstone and Baillière Tindall, and to the Editor of the *British Journal of Obstetrics and Gynaecology* for permission to use previously published photographs.

Introductory Guide to Lesions

RED LESIONS

Bartholin's abscess
cellulitis
eczema
erythrasma
extramammary Paget's disease
folliculitis
gonorrhoea in a child
hidradenitis
infection superimposed on dermatoses or trauma
lichen sclerosus
lichen simplex
lichenification
psoriasis
tinea
vestibulitis
vulval intra-epithelial neoplasia
vulvitis, e.g. candidosis, trichomoniasis

PALE/WHITE LESIONS

lichen sclerosus
lichen simplex
lichenification
postinflammatory hypopigmentation
vitiligo
vulval intra-epithelial neoplasia

PIGMENTED LESIONS

Melanocytic
lentigo
malignant melanoma
mole

Non-melanocytic
basal cell carcinoma
HPV lesions
post-inflammatory hyperpigmentation
seborrhoeic wart
vulval intra-epithelial neoplasia

Haemosiderin
caruncle
lichen sclerosus
prolapse
vestibulitis

PAPULES

chancre
condylomata lata
Fox–Fordyce disease
granuloma inguinale (donovanosis)
HPV lesions
lichen planus
lichen sclerosus
lymphangiectasia
lymphogranuloma venereum
molluscum contagiosum
vestibular papillae
vulval intra-epithelial neoplasia

TUMOURS

Benign neoplasms
haemangioma
seborrhoeic wart
skin tag

Malignant neoplasms
basal cell carcinoma
malignant melanoma
squamous cell carcinoma

PSEUDOTUMOURS

cysts
condylomata lata
endometrioma

ULCERS, BLISTERS, ERODED LESIONS

amoebiasis
aphthous ulcers
Behçet's syndrome
bullous disorders
chancre
chancroid
fixed drug eruption
granuloma inguinale (donovanosis)
herpes simplex
herpes zoster
lichen planus (eroded)
lichen sclerosus (eroded)
mucous patches
pyoderma gangrenosum
synergistic bacterial gangrene
ulcerated tumours
vestibulitis
vulval intra-epithelial neoplasia

OEDEMA

With scarring
chronic infection, e.g. granuloma inguinale
(donovanosis),
hidradenitis
lymphogranuloma venereum

Without scarring
Acute
Bartholin's abscess
candidosis
cellulitis
contact dermatitis
synergistic bacterial gangrene

Chronic
idiopathic
secondary to cellulitis (repeated)
secondary to infection, e.g. filariasis
secondary to inflammatory bowel disease
secondary to radiotherapy
secondary to surgery

SCARRING

cicatricial pemphigoid
hidradenitis
following infection: granuloma inguinale
(donovanosis), lymphogranuloma venereum
radiotherapy
surgery
trauma

MISCELLANEOUS

anatomical variants, e.g. ambiguous genitalia
other congenital defects
circumcision
pediculosis
varicose veins

LESIONS OF THE URETHRA

Infective
HPV
HSV

Neoplasms
benign
malignant

Pseudotumours
caruncle
prolapse

LESIONS OF THE VESTIBULE

Infective
abscesses of Bartholin's gland
HPV
HSV

Neoplasms of Bartholin's gland
benign
malignant

Pseudotumours
cyst of Bartholin's gland
mucinous cyst

Dermatological disorders
aphthous ulcers
Behçet's syndrome
cicatricial pemphigoid
lichen planus
lichen sclerosus
pemphigus
Stevens–Johnson syndrome
toxic epidermal necrolysis
vestibular papillomatosis
vestibulitis

SYMPTOMS

Symptoms are less reliable than signs. They depend
on the patient's personality, sensibility and ability to
express herself. They should never be given undue
diagnostic importance. However, some conditions do
typically tend to itch or to burn and, with the caveat
above, the following groupings are of some general
validity:

Pruritus (itching)

Infections
candidosis
warts

Any dermatological condition
especially eczema, lichen simplex, lichen sclerosus
and psoriasis.

Neoplasia
squamous cell carcinoma
tumours in general
VIN

Pain, soreness, burning

Infections
herpes simplex
herpes zoster
Trichomonas infection

Any dermatological condition
especially eczema, lichen planus (erosive), lichen simplex, lichen sclerosus, psoriasis

Vulvodynia
All variants (see Appendix B).

Trauma

Superficial dyspareunia

This may accompany any inflammatory lesion but when given as a specific main complaint it usually reflects either vulval vestibulitis, or lichen sclerosus with involvement of the perineum and/or fourchette.

1. General Principles

The clinician must be familiar with the appearance of the normal vulva (Fig. 1.1). A careful, systematic examination of the vulva should be carried out under good light conditions, using a magnifying glass if necessary. A diagram is useful for recording findings and photography is a valuable adjunct for records and teaching purposes.

Although colposcopy, which provides further light and magnification, is invaluable for study of the cervix and vagina, it is of somewhat limited value for the vulva. It can help in delineation and follow-up of lesions such as vulval intra-epithelial neoplasia (VIN) (Fig. 1.2), and in directing biopsy, but it is not a substitute for histological examination. Toluidine blue and acetic acid are sometimes used in conjunction with colposcopy (Fig. 1.3):

1. Toluidine blue stains widened intercellular spaces and nuclei. It will pick out neoplasia but may give false-positive results in eroded areas (Fig. 1.4).
2. Acetic acid produces an essentially non-specific whitening (light reflection), which can be helpful in delineating warts or VIN but which can mislead if its whiteness is taken to signify the invariable

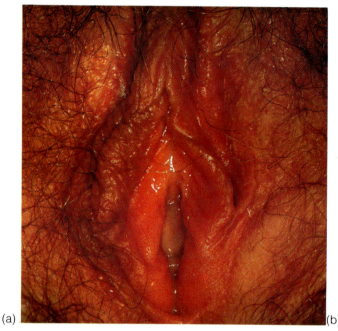

(a)

Fig. 1.1 (a) The normal vulva.

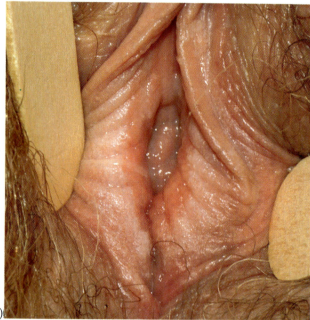

(b)

(b) Hart's line: a natural demarcation between the labia minora and the limits of the vestibule, seen more easily in some patients than in others.

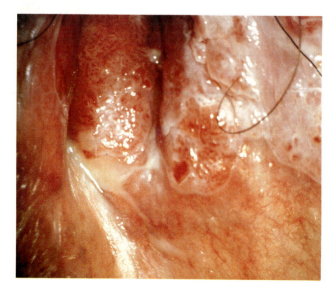

Fig. 1.2 Appearance of an area of VIN with foci of invasive carcinoma. Abnormal vascular pattern.

presence of such lesions, for example in papillomatosis of the vestibule (Fig. 1.5).

Histology will usually be required. In some cases this will follow upon excision, in others it will be sought in biopsy specimens that may need to be multiple and to be repeated. Punch biopsy, using a disposable Keyes punch, is the favourite method for outpatients (Fig. 1.6). Local anaesthesia with 1 or 2% lignocaine is suitable. The application of a eutectic mixture of prilocaine and lignocaine (Emla cream) for 10–15 min prior to biopsy, the thighs being kept close together to provide natural occlusion, helps by rendering insertion of the needle painless (and, in very superficial intervention, e.g. curettage or snipping of condylomata acuminata, can suffice in itself to furnish adequate anaesthesia). Various sizes of the biopsy punch are available. A 4 mm punch is usually used. Haemostasis can be with cautery or a silver nitrate stick and a stitch may occasionally be required, particularly with a 6 mm punch. It is important to obtain a specimen that is appropriately deep.

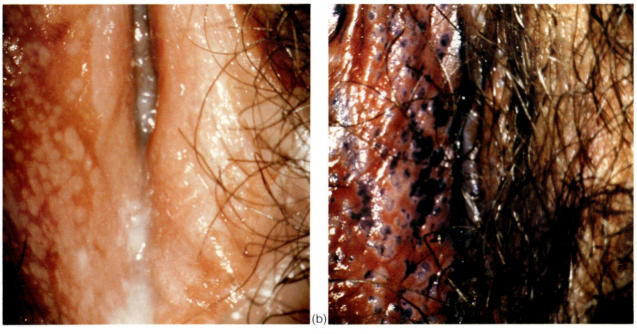

(a) (b)

Fig. 1.3 Area of epithelium. (a) Acetowhite appearance. **(b)** With toluidine blue applied.

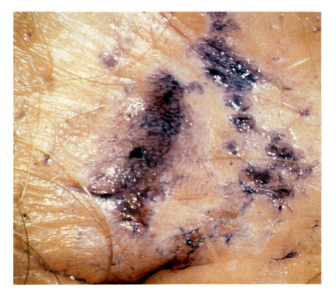

Fig. 1.4 False-positive reaction to toluidine blue in an area that was eroded but not malignant.

Specimens for immunofluorescence in the bullous diseases must be perilesional. The tissue removed must either be sent to the laboratory at once in liquid nitrogen or (after washing with saline) put into special transport medium, which can then be sent through the post. Where infections are suspected, further measures are required.

Many pathogens reach the vulva through sexual contact – pediculosis pubis, trichomoniasis, gonorrhoea, chancroid, donovanosis, syphilis, chlamydial infection, genital herpes, papilloma virus infection and molluscum contagiosum are all introduced in this way. The presence of any one of these infections indicates the possible presence of others and it is important that screening tests for the common sexually transmitted diseases (STDs) should be performed. These should include:

1. Microscopy and/or culture for *Trichomonas vaginalis*.
2. Cervical culture for *Neisseria gonorrhoeae*.
3. Cervical culture, or an antigen detection test, for *Chlamydia trachomatis*.
4. Serological tests for syphilis.

If the presence of an STD is proved, examination of the male sex partner is necessary, both for his own benefit and to prevent to-and-fro infection.

Other vulval infections, e.g. schistosomiasis, candidosis, *Tinea cruris*, infection by pyogenic cocci and herpes zoster, are not sexually transmitted. Tests for associated infections and contact tracing are not necessary for women with these conditions.

In all cases the cause of a vulval infection should be established by appropriate laboratory tests, so that the correct antimicrobial therapy can be arranged.

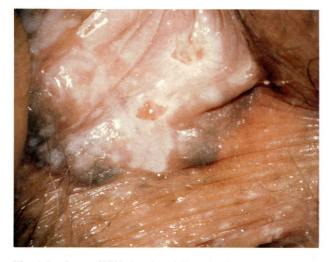

Fig. 1.5 Area of VIN showing delineation by acetowhite appearance.

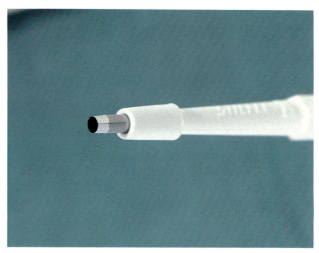

Fig. 1.6 Disposable biopsy punches are available in various diameters: the 4 mm is used most often.

2. Infections

PEDICULOSIS PUBIS

Pediculosis pubis is a common sexually transmitted disease caused by the crab louse – *Phthirus pubis*. This wingless insect, which is flattened dorsoventrally and 1–2 mm long, has two of its six legs modified for grasping hair (Fig. 2.1) and adult lice feed by sucking blood from their hosts. The eggs (nits) are cemented to hairs near the hair roots (Fig. 2.2). The incubation period is about 4 weeks. Infestation may be symptomless but patients usually present with irritation, or because they have seen the insects moving. In women the pubic, vulval and peri-anal areas are most often affected and adult lice and nits may be present (Fig. 2.3). Non-genital hairy areas such as the axillae, eyebrows and eyelashes may also be affected.

Tests for other STDs should be performed before treatment. After bathing or showering, 0.5% malathion lotion should be applied to all hairy areas except the scalp. The medication is washed off after 24 hours, when the clothes and bed linen should be changed. Patients should be warned that the nits may persist for a while after treatment, but that they are dead. Sex partners should receive the same treatment.

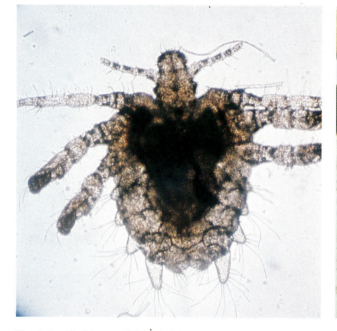

Fig. 2.1 *Phthirus pubis*: **adult female.**

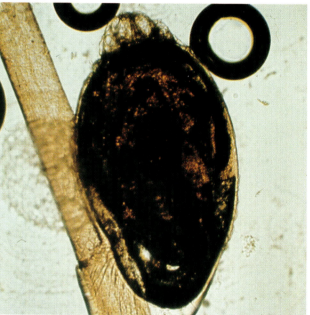

Fig. 2.2 *Phthirus pubis*: **nit.** The ovum is firmly attached to the hair by its chitinous coat.

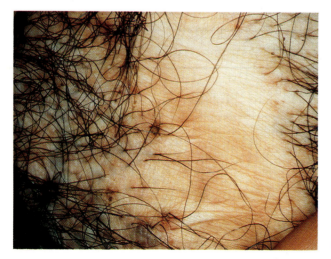

Fig. 2.3 **Pediculosis pubis.** Showing pediculi and nits.

FILARIASIS

Filariasis is caused by filarial worms, either *Wucheria bancrofti or Brugia malayi*. Bancroftian filariasis is the most widespread human filarial infection, occurring mostly in Asia (India, Indonesia and China), although it is also common in Bangladesh, Thailand, tropical parts of East, Central and West Africa, parts of South America, Central America and in some of the West Indies. Brugian filariasis is more restricted in distribution (China, India, Indonesia, Malaysia and Thailand) and there is no definite proof that it causes genital lesions.

The larvae are inoculated into human blood by mosquitoes and develop into microfilaria in the lymphatic vessels. They cause inflammation that, if it occurs in inguinal glands, gives rise to genital lymphoedema and elephantiasis. Lymphoedema affects the vulva bilaterally, although the swelling is often more marked on one side. Biopsy of affected lymph nodes may confirm the diagnosis if histology shows dead filaria, but the appearances are often non-specific. The condition must be distinguished from other causes of lymphatic obstruction with vulval swelling, e.g. lymphogranuloma venereum, carcinoma and tuberculosis (Fig. 2.4). Treatment is with diethyl-carbamazine, increasing from 1 mg/kg/day to 6 mg/kg/day in divided doses over 3 days and continued for 3 weeks.

SCHISTOSOMIASIS

Three species of the genus *Schistosoma* infect humans, causing schistosomiasis, which occasionally affects the genital tract. *S. japonicum* occurs only in the Orient but *S. mansoni* and *S. haematobium* are more widespread. *S. haematobium*, which is the most likely to affect the female genital tract, is common in the Middle East, particularly in Egypt, Iraq, Tunisia and Algeria.

The fluke larvae enter the bloodstream through cuts and fissures in the skin during wading or swimming. Females mature in the portal veins and, after copulation, migrate to the pelvic venous plexus, where they lay eggs that eventually work their way back to the skin. The eggs are shed into water where they infect their intermediate host—a snail.

The developing flukes may cause granulomatous lesions first in the labia majora, then in other parts of the vulva; haematuria may also occur. The disease is very persistent and ulceration and scarring may occur (Fig. 2.5).

Schistosomiasis must be distinguished from condylomata acuminata, lymphogranuloma venereum and vulval carcinoma. The diagnosis is best established by biopsy; ova also being found in the urine, faeces or vaginal discharge.

A single oral dose of praziquantel 40 mg/kg is usually curative.

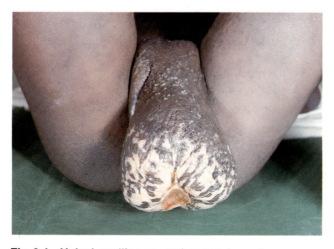

Fig. 2.4 Vulval swelling secondary to tuberculous inguinal adenitis.

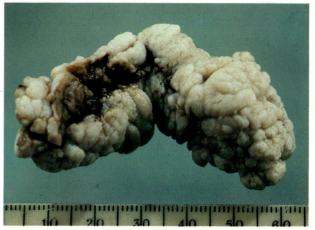

Fig. 2.5 Schistosomiasis. Excised granulomatous vulval tissue. Histology of these active lesions shows ova surrounded by an intense inflammatory reaction.

TRICHOMONAS VAGINALIS

Trichomonas vaginalis is a protozoon that specifically infects the genital tract. It is sexually transmitted and may be carried asymptomatically in both men and women. The duration of infestation is usually prolonged in women and as many as half the women infected with this organism are asymptomatic.

The symptoms vary from a minimal, often yellow–green, vaginal discharge to a profuse, purulent, frothy discharge, visible externally, and an inflamed vaginal and vulval mucosae. In a small number of cases the cervix is inflamed with punctate haemorrhages—a 'strawberry cervix' (Fig. 2.6). In more severe cases the profuse discharge may cause a perivulval rash with irritation and associated oedema (Fig. 2.7).

Diagnosis should be made by microscopy of a wet mount of vaginal secretions. The organism can be identified as it moves using its undulating membrane and motile flagellae (Fig. 2.8). The organism may be cultured and can be seen on a Papanicolaou stain of cells on cervical cytology.

Metronidazole is the most effective drug and may be given as a 2 g single dose or as 400 mg twice a day for 5 days. However, metronidazole-resistant strains of *T. vaginalis* have been reported.

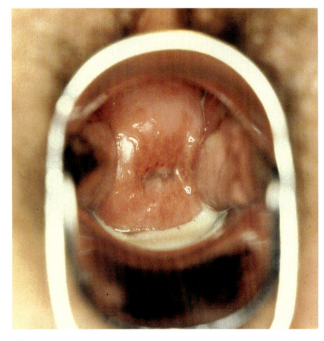

Fig. 2.6   Trichomoniasis. Profuse yellow discharge with punctate haemorrhages on the cervix ('strawberry' cervix).

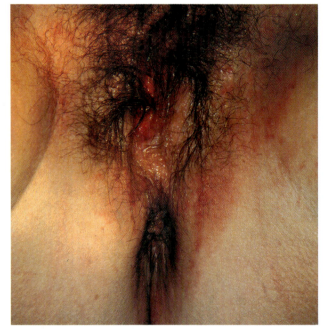

Fig. 2.7   Trichomoniasis. Vulvitis with perivulval rash.

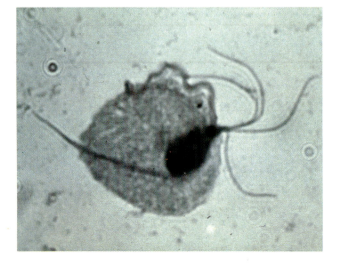

Fig. 2.8   Trichomoniasis. Microscopy of wet mount showing *Trichomonas vaginalis*. Note the four flagellae and lateral undulating membrane.

AMOEBIASIS

Entamoeba histolytica can cause cutaneous lesions and gastro-intestinal symptoms. It exists in two forms, the motile trophozoite and the cyst. The cysts can be transmitted directly through oro-anal contact or indirectly via fomites. The lesions may occur by direct extension from the bowel but are most common after surgical treatment in patients with an infected bowel.

Genital lesions affecting the vulva, perineum and cervix are an unusual complication of this very common infection. *E. histolytica* is found world-wide but is particularly common in tropical and subtropical countries.

The lesions begin as cutaneous abscesses, which have a central necrotic zone with a purulent exudate.

They develop an undermined margin and erythematous halo (Fig. 2.9). The ulcers are irregular but sharply defined with a sloughing base (Fig. 2.10). They are very painful and may be destructive; there may be associated local lymphadenopathy. The condition should be distinguished from deep mycosis, early syphilis (see p. 21), lymphogranuloma venereum (see p. 23) and donovanosis (see p. 20).

The trophozoite of *E. histolytica* can be found in the purulent exudate from the ulcers. Histologically, the trophozoite may be seen with a surrounding inflammatory reaction (Fig. 2.11). Metronidazole, 600 mg three times a day for 5 days is an effective treatment. Bowel disease is always associated and a course of diloxanide furoate should follow the metronidazole to clear the cysts from the bowel.

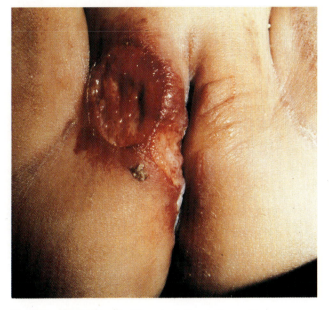

Fig. 2.9 Amoebiasis. Sharply defined ulcer with undermined margin in a child.

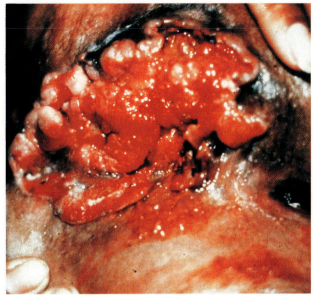

Fig. 2.10 Amoebiasis. Large ulcer with sloughing base.

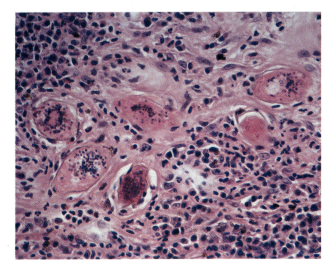

Fig. 2.11 Amoebiasis. Trophozoites staining red (PAS × 100).

13

CANDIDOSIS (THRUSH)

Vulvovaginal yeast infection is common. *Candida albicans* causes 90 per cent of vaginal infections with other *Candida* species causing the remainder. Only *Candida albicans* produces hyphae in culture (Fig. 2.12).

Endogenous yeasts are ubiquitous, colonizing the gastro-intestinal tract, skin, mouth and vagina; symptoms occur when this flora overgrows. The causes of symptomatic yeast infection are not completely understood but pregnancy, diabetes, immunosuppression and systemic antimicrobial therapy are recognized predisposing factors, although no predisposing factors are identified in some cases of recurrent candidal vulvovaginitis.

The cardinal symptom of candidosis is pruritus, which usually affects the labia and vulva. Swelling of the labia and superficial dyspareunia may occur. There may be genital odour. The vulva is erythematous and excoriated with accompanying labial oedema (Fig. 2.13). A rash may be present in the genital area involving the perineum and peri-anal region and satellite lesions may be seen. Fissuring of the skin may occur (Figs 2.14 and 2.15), especially in women suffering from eczema or lichen sclerosus, and there

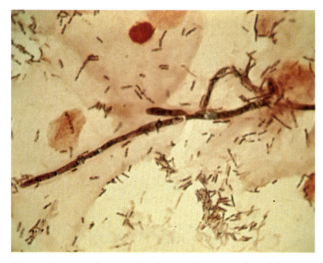

Fig. 2.12 Candidosis. Hyphae and spore of *Candida albicans* in vaginal smear. Gram stain.

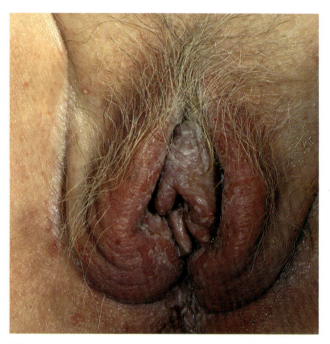

Fig. 2.13 Candidosis. Severe vulvitis due to *Candida albicans*. Note vulval oedema, rash extending to the peri-anal region and satellite lesions.

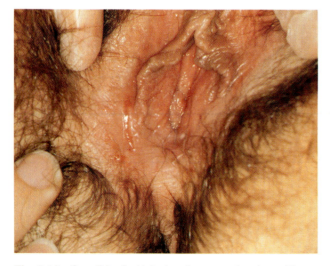

Fig. 2.14 Candidosis. Vulval erythema and oedema. There are linear fissures on the labia.

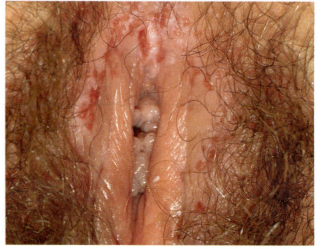

Fig. 2.15 Candidosis. Linear fissures, in which *Candida* was found in a patient with lichen sclerosus and herpes simplex virus.

may be superficial ulceration. In long-standing infections, the skin may become glazed and atrophic-looking. The vagina may be erythematous with adherent white plaque. The discharge may be thick and curdy or thin with white flecks.

Candidosis may co-exist with other genital infections, and the clinical picture may be confused with herpetic infection and other causes of vaginitis, e.g. *Trichomonas vaginalis*. Other causes of vaginal infection should be excluded, e.g. bacterial vaginosis.

Vaginal yeast infection may be diagnosed by microscopy in 50 per cent of patients with a wet preparation in normal saline or mixed with 10% potassium hydroxide and warmed. A vaginal smear may be stained by Gram's method. Culture of yeasts on Sabouraud's medium is more sensitive. The urine should be tested to exclude glycosuria.

Symptomatic candidosis requires treatment. Local antifungal therapy can be given in the form of imidazole pessaries (e.g. clotrimazole for a 1-, 3- or 6-day course) or polyene pessaries (e.g. nystatin for 14 days). Systemic single-dose oral therapy with fluconazole 150 mg has recently been shown to be safe and effective. Other practical measures, e.g. saline bathing and avoiding tight clothing, nylon underwear and perfumed toiletries, may decrease the duration of symptoms and help prevent recurrences.

TINEA CRURIS

Tinea cruris is seen more often in men than women. The usual cause is *Trichophyton rubrum* or *Epidermophyton floccosum*.

Tinea presents as an erythematous plaque, which spreads peripherally and tends to clear in the centre (Figs 2.16 and 2.17). The infection may spread to involve the vulva, perineum and peri-anal areas. There is often a focus of infection elsewhere, for example on the feet.

The differential diagnosis includes cutaneous candidosis, although the lesions of the latter are often more inflamed. It may be confused with erythrasma but this has a brownish colour and fluoresces orange–red in Wood's light. Other non-infective skin conditions, e.g. flexural psoriasis, should be considered in the differential diagnosis.

This condition is diagnosed by microscopy of scrapings from the edge of the lesions suspended in 10% potassium hydroxide when fungal filaments are seen. The clinical material can also be sent for culture. Local application of an imidazole cream, e.g. clotrimazole twice daily, clears the infection in 4–6 weeks. A course of systemic griseofulvin is justified in severe cases.

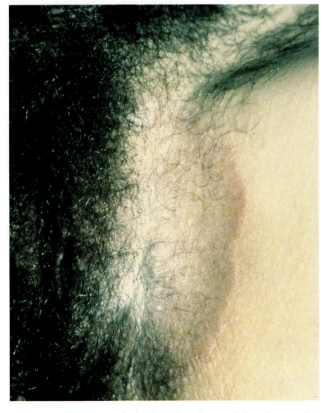

Fig. 2.16 *Tinea cruris.* Lesion showing peripheral spread.

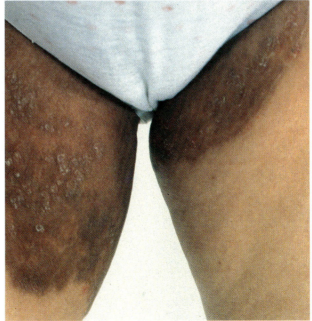

Fig. 2.17 *Tinea cruris.* Typical lesion extending down the thighs.

PYOGENIC INFECTIONS

Staphylococcus aureus may cause vulval folliculitis (Fig. 2.18) and abscesses following minor trauma such as

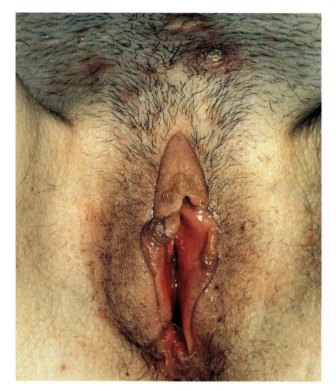

Fig. 2.18 Folliculitis of the vulva.

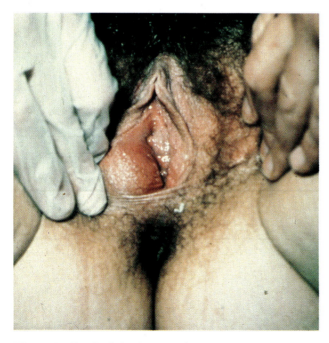

Fig. 2.19 Bartholin's abscess. Such lesions are usually caused by either pyogenic cocci or *N. gonorrhoeae*. Surgical treatment is necessary.

shaving. It may complicate almost any vulval infection or dermatosis, including warts, molluscum contagiosum and ulcerative conditions. *S. aureus* is a common cause of infection of Bartholin's duct (Fig. 2.19), which may also be caused by *N. gonorrhoeae*, *Escherichia coli* and *Streptococcus faecalis*.

The clinical features of infection of Bartholin's duct are similar whatever its aetiology. It may be secondary to a previously existing cyst or it may arise *de novo*. The area becomes swollen and tender and the opening of the duct is infected; it may be possible to express purulent matter from the duct. Severe pain, with surrounding erythema and oedema, accompanies the development of an abscess. The abscess often discharges spontaneously but recurrent infection, with or without the formation of a cyst, is common. Rupture of a Bartholin's abscess occasionally leaves a fistulous opening between one part of the vulva and another, which prevents further recurrences (Fig. 2.20).

Streptococcus pyogenes may cause vulval erysipelas — a spreading inflammation of the dermis that causes pain, redness and swelling. Fissures, minor injuries and underlying skin diseases, especially lichen sclerosus in children, are predisposing factors. The condition is also a hazard where there is some degree of lymphatic obstruction, e.g. following vulvectomy.

Ideally, the nature of the infecting organism should be determined by bacteriological examination of pus from the infected area. Urethral and cervical specimens for culture for *N. gonorrhoeae* should also be collected. In practice, an acute infection may require treatment before laboratory results are available and a presumptive clinical diagnosis of the nature of the infecting organism has to be made.

Severe furunculosis or folliculitis, presumed or

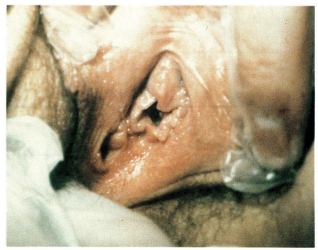

Fig. 2.20 Vulval fistula following the spontaneous rupture of Bartholin's abscess.

known to be due to *S. aureus*, is treated with fluclox-acillin 250 mg four times a day for 7 days. Mild infections hardly require antibiotic therapy. Oral or parenteral penicillin is very effective against strepto-coccal infection.

Early infections of Bartholin's duct may respond to antimicrobial drugs but an abscess will require drain-age under general anaesthesia. Marsupialization of the abscess or cyst should be performed as soon as practicable to prevent recurrent infections.

GONORRHOEA

Gonorrhoea is a highly infectious sexually transmitted disease, predominantly infecting anogenital mucosae. It is caused by *Neisseria gonorrhoeae*, a Gram-negative diplococcus, which grows well on special media.

Gonorrhoea is the most common STD in the world and is particularly common in developing countries. It is highly infectious; the risk of a woman contracting gonorrhoea from a single sexual contact with an infected man is about 75 per cent. *N. gonorrhoeae* can be transmitted to a baby during delivery and may cause ophthalmia neonatorum, a potentially blinding eye infection.

N. gonorrhoeae infects the cervix, urethra and rectum during intercourse and the pharynx during fellatio. The incubation period is 2–5 days. About 50 per cent of these infections are symptomless, the remainder pre-sent with vaginal discharge, dysuria, lower abdominal discomfort, acute abdominal pain or systemic illness. Many cases of gonorrhoea in women are accompanied by trichomoniasis or chlamydial infection.

Examination may show that pus can be expressed from the urethra (Fig. 2.21) or from the ducts of Skene's para-urethral glands or Bartholin's glands. A speculum examination often reveals mucopurulent cervicitis and there may be a purulent vaginal dis-charge from associated trichomoniasis.

The complications of gonorrhoea include peri-urethral abscess (Fig. 2.22) and Bartholin's abscess, but the most serious are disseminated gonococcal infection and acute salpingitis, which develop in about 15 per cent of women.

Specimens for microscopy and culture should be collected from all potentially infected sites—the urethra, cervix, anorectum and pharynx. High vaginal swabs are insensitive and should not be used. Speci-mens for culture are sent to the laboratory in Stuart's transport medium. Examination of Gram-stained smears for intracellular Gram-negative diplococci is quick but less sensitive than culture; microscopy of rectal or pharyngeal specimens is useless.

In areas where *N. gonorrhoeae* is sensitive to penicil-lin, 3 g oral amoxycillin plus 1 g oral probenecid may be given. If the organism is resistant to penicillin (as are the majority outside Europe) cefotaxime 1.0 g, or spectinomycin 2.0 g, given intramuscularly, are satis-factory.

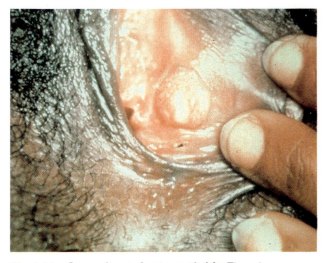

Fig. 2.21 Gonorrhoea. Acute urethritis. The urinary meatus is oedematous and there is a purulent exudate.

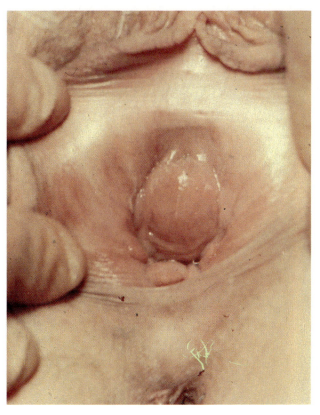

Fig. 2.22 Gonorrhoea. Peri-urethral abscess. This is an unusual complication.

ERYTHRASMA

Erythrasma is caused by infection with *Corynebacterium minutissimum*. This organism forms part of the normal skin flora but may overgrow and cause a rash, particularly in warm humid conditions.

Genital erythrasma affects the groins and natal cleft, where it causes an itchy rash of red–brown scaly patches (Fig. 2.23). Examination under Wood's light shows a coral-red fluorescence.

Erythrasma must be differentiated from *Tinea cruris*, intertrigo, flexural eczema and seborrhoeic dermatitis. The use of Wood's light is useful but *C. minutissimum* can be cultured from skin scrapings on appropriate media.

Erythromycin 250 mg four times a day for 2 weeks is effective, as is topical clotrimazole, used as necessary.

CHANCROID

Chancroid, or soft sore, is an acute sexually transmitted infection characterized by one or more genital ulcers and often accompanied by painful inguinal lymphadenopathy. It is very common in some tropical areas (Africa, South East Asia, Central America and the Pacific) but outbreaks have occurred in Western industrialized countries.

Haemophilus ducreyi is the causative organism. The disease has a short incubation period, averaging 3–6 days. The initial lesion is a transient papule, which rapidly progresses to an ulcer. The ulcer may have a round edge but is usually irregular, with a red margin and a sloughy granular base (Fig. 2.24). Lesions may be single or multiple (Fig. 2.25) and adjacent lesions tend to become confluent. They are painful and most are deep and excavated into the skin. Chancroidal ulcers are commonly found in women at sites prone to trauma during sexual intercourse – the labia, fourchette, perineum and peri-anal areas (Fig. 2.26). The prevalence of chancroid is greater in men than women. This may be explained by the occurrence of small asymptomatic lesions in women (Fig. 2.27) and the presence of vaginal and cervical ulcers.

Inguinal lymphadenopathy occurs 1–2 weeks after the genital lesion in about half the cases; occasionally it may be the presenting feature. The enlarged glands may be unilateral or bilateral. A mass of glands may become matted together (chancroidal bubo) and progress to form abscesses, which then rupture.

The major differential diagnoses include syphilis, genital herpes, lymphogranuloma venereum and secondarily infected traumatic lesions. Chancroid may co-exist with other causes of genital ulceration and it is important to exclude these by appropriate laboratory tests. It is essential to perform syphilis serology on all patients with genital ulceration and/or lymphadenopathy.

Laboratory diagnosis depends on the isolation of *H. ducreyi* from the ulcers or from the pus from bubos. Microscopy of stained smears is difficult to interpret.

H. ducreyi has developed resistance to penicillins, sulphonamides and tetracyclines. Recommended treatment is erythromycin (500 mg four times a day) or trimethoprim and sulphamethoxazole (160 mg and 800 mg, respectively, twice a day) for 7–10 days. Abscesses should be aspirated.

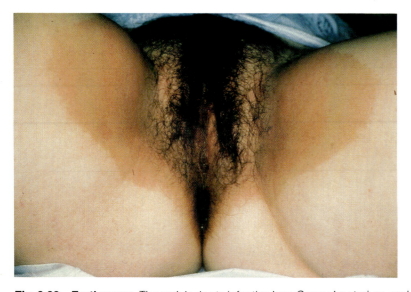

Fig. 2.23 Erythrasma. The rash is due to infection by a *Corynebacterium*, and rapidly regresses with oral erythromycin therapy or topical clotrimazole.

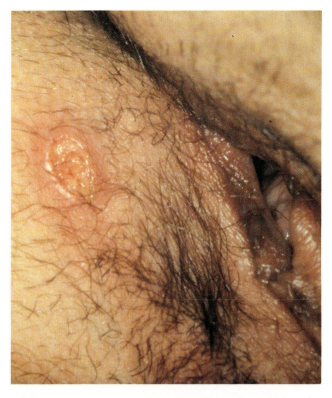

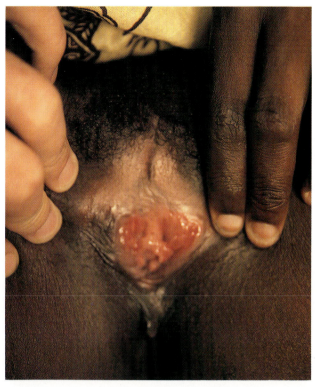

Fig. 2.24 Chancroid. Single ulcer with a round edge and granular base.

Fig. 2.25 Chancroid. Multiple ulcers visible on labia minora.

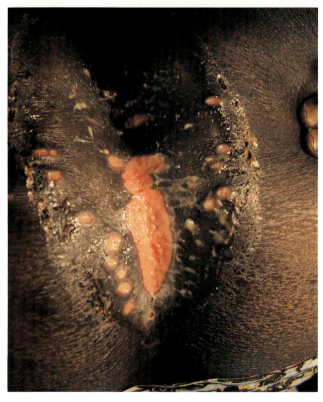

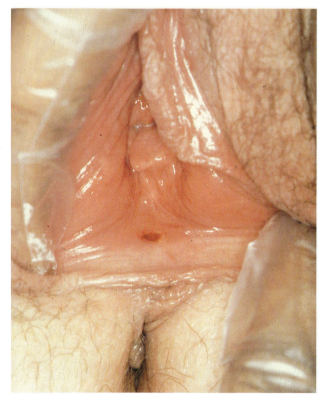

Fig. 2.26 Chancroid. Many small ulcers and one large ulcer in the peri-anal region.

Fig. 2.27 Chancroid. Small ulcer at the posterior fourchette. It was asymptomatic.

GRANULOMA INGUINALE (DONOVANOSIS)

Granuloma inguinale is a slowly progressive ulcerative disease of the genitalia caused by the bacterium *Calymmatobacterium granulomatis*. This is a Gram-negative encapsulated rod that has not been grown *in vitro*. *C. granulomatis* is of low infectivity and is presumed to be spread by sexual contact through skin abrasions. It occurs in tropical regions in people with poor hygiene (India, Brazil, the West Indies and West Africa).

The incubation period is usually 2–3 weeks and the initial presentation is of one or more indurated papules. In women these occur on the labia, fourchette and mons veneris. The papules ulcerate irregularly and eventually may involve a large area, including the perineum and anus (Fig. 2.28). The ulcers have a beefy red granular base and usually have a rolled edge (Figs 2.29a and 2.29b). Regional lymphadenopathy does not occur but the granulomatous lesions may extend subcutaneously and be mistaken for lymph gland involvement (pseudobubo). Vulval granulation may extend into the vagina and late complications include strictures of the urethra, vagina or anus. Healing is uncommon without treatment and the granulated area may become secondarily infected or undergo neoplastic change.

The diagnosis depends on demonstrating the organism ('Donovan bodies') (Fig. 2.30) in tissue smears. Specimens are obtained by biopsy or curet-

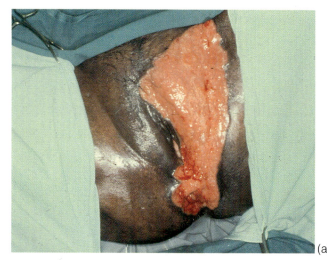

Fig. 2.28   Granuloma inguinale (donovanosis). Extensive area of ulceration requiring surgical debridement in a woman with long-standing infection.

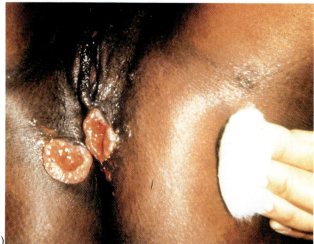

(a)

Fig. 2.29a   Granuloma inguinale (donovanosis). Diescrete perineal ulcers demonstrating the typical rolled edge and granular base.

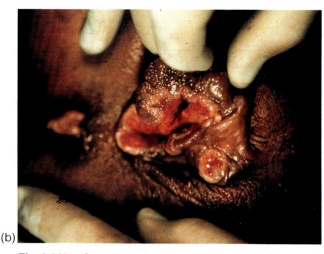

(b)

Fig. 2.29b   Granuloma inguinale (donovanosis). Confluent ulceration with irregular edges.

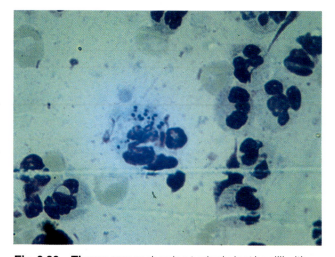

Fig. 2.30   Tissue smear showing typical giant bacilli with rounded ends (Donovan bodies) within neutrophils and macrophages (Giemsa stain).

tings and are stained with Warthin–Starry or Giemsa stains. The lesions may mimic those of primary and secondary syphilis, so syphilis serology is essential.

Many antibiotics have been used for treatment with varying efficacy. Possibilities include tetracycline hydrochloride 500 mg orally four times a day for at least 10 days and ampicillin 500 mg four times a day for 2 weeks.

SYPHILIS

Syphilis is a chronic systemic sexually transmitted disease caused by *Treponema pallidum*, a slender spiral organism 6–15 μm × 0.25 μm. In a fresh wet preparation it can be seen to undergo rotary movements and angulation. The organism cannot be cultured on artificial media but stocks may be maintained by inoculation into rabbits' testicles.

Acquired syphilis in adults is a sexually transmitted disease; intra-uterine infection of a fetus may result in fetal death or the birth of a baby with signs of congenital syphilis. In Europe and North America the incidence of syphilis in women is low, but it is a common disease in developing countries.

After an incubation period of 9–90 days the initial lesion—the primary chancre—appears. This begins as a small papule, which enlarges to form an indurated ulcer up to 1 cm in diameter. Chancres are usually, but not invariably, painless, and are multiple in 15 per cent of cases. In women they appear on the fourchette or other parts of the vulva, and less often at the anus, perigenital sites and on the cervix (Figs 2.31—2.33). In most cases regional lymphadenopathy develops within a week of the appearance of the chancre; the nodes are rubbery and painless. Without treatment, primary chancres heal in up to 6 weeks.

Secondary syphilis appears 3–6 weeks after the primary chancre. This is a systemic disease. The main signs are skin rashes, mucosal ulceration, generalized adenopathy and general malaise. Several kinds of lesion are seen on the vulva. Condylomata lata are usually perivulval and peri-anal (Figs 2.34 and 2.35). They are soft and spongy, with flat tops that may become eroded. Mucous patches are painless, eroded

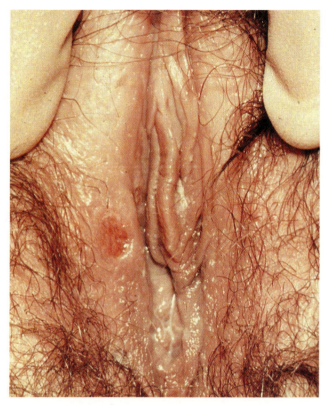

Fig. 2.31 Syphilis. Primary chancre of the labium majus.
The ulcer is indurated and usually painless.

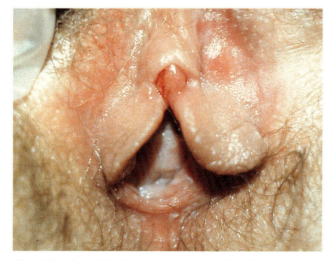

Fig. 2.32 Syphilis. Primary chancre of the clitoris.
A lesion of this sort may escape detection.

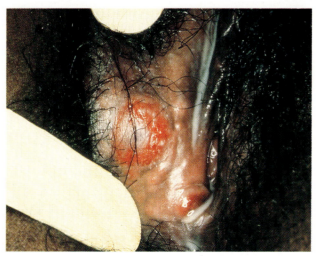

Fig. 2.33 Syphilis. Primary chancre of the labium minus.

21

areas affecting the labia minor and other moist sites. Any of the skin rashes of secondary syphilis—macular, papular, papulosquamous or pustular—can appear on the vulva.

With exacerbations and remissions, secondary syphilis can last for up to 2 years, but eventually all signs of disease disappear, although the patient is still infected with *T. pallidum*—this is latent syphilis.

Late syphilis—gummatous disease, cardiovascular syphilis and neurosyphilis—develops in about one-third of these patients within 5–20 years. Gummas of the vulva—nodular and/or ulcerative lesions—are very rare today.

In early congenital syphilis, bullous or papulo-squamous lesions may appear on the baby's vulva as part of the syphilitic dermatosis. Condylomata lata may develop later.

Chancres of the vulva must be differentiated from other ulcerative lesions—genital herpes, chancroid, lymphogranuloma venereum, donovanosis, pyogenic lesions, Behçet's syndrome and carcinoma. The vulval lesions of secondary syphilis may resemble many dermatoses and, in particular, condylomata lata may be confused with condylomata acuminata.

The laboratory diagnosis of early syphilis depends on the dark-field examination of serum expressed from the lesions or obtained by gland puncture. *T. pallidum* is extremely difficult to identify in smears

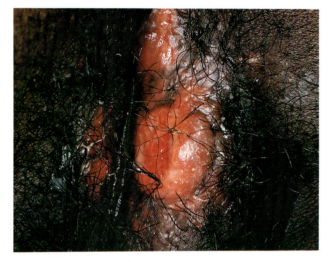

Fig. 2.34 Secondary syphilis. Condylomata lata. These flat-topped lesions are highly contagious. They must not be mistaken for genital warts (condylomata acuminata).

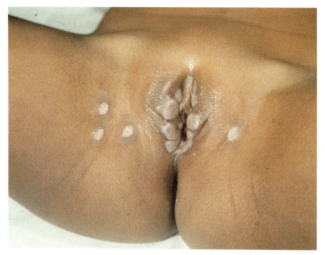

Fig. 2.35 Secondary syphilis. Condylomata lata in a child.

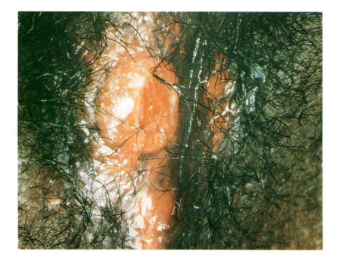

Fig. 2.36 Syphilis. The same lesion as in Fig. 2.33, photographed 48 h after the first injection of penicillin. The Jarisch–Herxheimer reaction has caused temporary enlargement of the chancre.

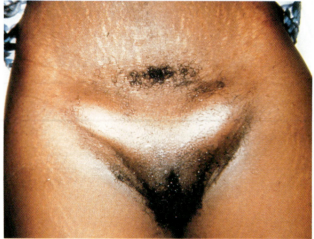

Fig. 2.37 Lymphogranuloma venereum. Bilateral inguinal lymphadenopathy. The primary vulval lesion is small and may go unnoticed. The glands are tender and later suppurate; chronic discharging sinuses develop.

stained with conventional stains but, if the smears are treated with an antitreponemal monoclonal antibody, it can be easily identified. Serological tests for syphilis should always be performed. The Venereal Disease Reference Laboratory (VDRL) or rapid plasma reagin (RPR) test is positive in 50–70 per cent of patients with primary syphilis and the fluorescent treponemal antibodies (FTA ABS) test in about 80 per cent. All serological tests are strongly positive in secondary syphilis.

Patients with early syphilis respond well to:

1. Daily intramuscular injection of procaine penicillin, 900 000 units, for 10 days.
2. Intramuscular injection of benzathine penicillin 2.4 mega units followed by a second injection of 2.4 mega units 1 week later.

Patients who are allergic to penicillin should be given tetracycline hydrochloride or oxytetracycline 2.0 g a day in divided doses for 2 weeks.

The patient often experiences fever and malaise a few hours after the first dose of antimicrobial for primary or secondary syphilis. A primary chancre may enlarge or secondary manifestations appear for the first time. This Jarisch–Herxheimer reaction subsides in a day or two, and is not repeated with subsequent doses of the antimicrobial (Fig. 2.36).

LYMPHOGRANULOMA VENEREUM

A sexually transmitted disease affecting lymphoid tissue and showing a variety of early and late manifestations, lymphogranuloma venereum (LGV) is caused by specific types of *Chlamydia trachomatis* — L1, 2 or 3.

LGV is endemic in east and west Africa, India, South America and the Caribbean. Sporadic cases are seen in Europe and North America.

The incubation period is 2–5 days. The initial lesion is a small painless papule, vesicle or ulcer. In women this is most commonly found at the fourchette, but it may also appear on the labia, vagina or cervix. The lesion may easily escape notice.

Characteristic lymphadenopathy develops several weeks after the primary lesion. If this is on the vulva, the inguinal glands become enlarged and painful; they often suppurate and form multiple sinuses (Figs 2.37 and 2.38). The disease is inherently chronic and even with treatment healing is slow, often with much scarring.

Women with late LGV show chronic lymphadenopathy, discharging sinuses and symptoms and signs of proctocolitis. Vulval elephantiasis with ulceration (esthiomène) is due to lymphatic obstruction (Fig. 2.39).

Early LGV must be distinguished from other causes of genital ulceration and lymphadenopathy. Syphilis serology must always be performed. A specific diagnosis of LGV may be obtained by cell culture of aspirated pus for *C. trachomatis* but this test is not widely available. The LGV complement fixation test is useful — a titre of >64 is regarded as confirmatory if characteristic symptoms and signs are present.

Tetracycline hydrochloride or oxytetracycline 2.0 g a day in divided doses is given for 2 weeks in the first instance, but this may have to be extended if the clinical response is slow. Erythromycin in the same dosage is an alternative for patients who cannot tolerate tetracyclines. Abscesses should be aspirated.

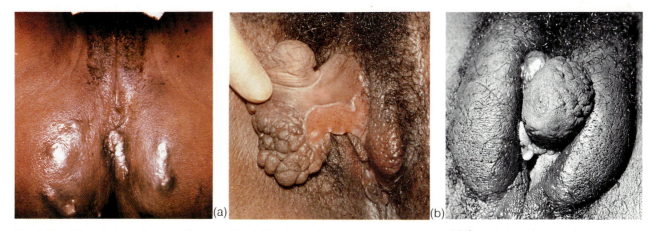

(a)　(b)

Fig. 2.38 Chronic lymphogranuloma venereum. These are multiple peri-anal sinuses with chronic inflammation and fibrosis.

Fig. 2.39 Lymphogranuloma venereum. (a) Chronic lymphogranuloma verereum, showing vulval elephantiasis with secondary ulceration (esthiomene). **(b)** Lymphoedema secondary to lymphogranuloma venereum.

GENITAL HERPES

The most common cause of genital ulcers in industrialized countries is herpes. This is a painful condition, which starts characteristically with erythematous lesions that become vesicular and then rupture to form shallow ulcers.

The virus responsible for this is herpes simplex virus (HSV). There are two virus types—HSV 1 causes predominantly oral herpes and HSV 2 genital herpes. However, there is good evidence that transmission may occur through orogenital contact as well as through genital contact, and the two types are not site-specific. During the initial skin infection the virus spreads along sensory nerves to the dorsal root ganglia, where it becomes latent. The virus may be reactivated to cause recurrence of the infection. This life-cycle has resulted in different clinical manifestations of genital herpes:

1. Primary genital herpes infection occurs approximately 1 week (range 2–12 days) after intimate contact with an infected person. Irritation at the site may occur before the appearance of a group of painful papules. The papules form vesicles (Fig. 2.40) and pustules, which then erode, particularly at sites of friction, to create superficial erosions (Fig. 2.41). These may crust and heal, but sometimes form ulcers. The lesions are usually small with an erythematous halo and surrounding oedema (Fig. 2.42).
2. Cervicitis is common in the primary attack (Fig. 2.43). The cervix may have discrete erosions or be red and friable. Associated symptoms may include dysuria and vaginal discharge.
3. Lesions may occur anywhere in the genital area, i.e. peri-anal and vulval; extragenital sites are occasionally involved. Painful inguinal lymphadenopathy is found in about 80 per cent of cases.

The presentation of primary genital herpes differs significantly between individuals according to host response. Chronic eczema renders the skin susceptible to more severe infection—eczema herpeticum (Fig. 2.44). In patients who have altered immunity, e.g. in

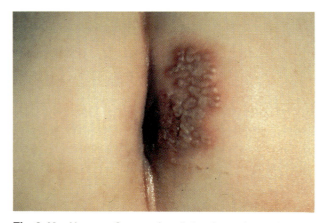

Fig. 2.40   Herpes. Group of vesicles due to herpes simplex virus type 2. Note the surrounding erythema.

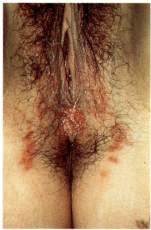

Fig. 2.41   Herpes. Multiple herpetic ulcers in a primary attack.

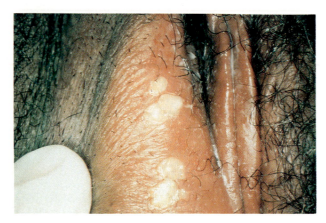

Fig. 2.42   Herpes. Typical herpetic ulcers on labia with surrounding oedema in a primary attack.

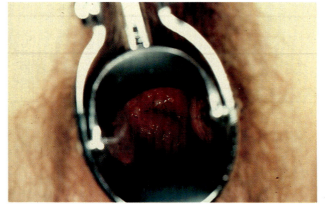

Fig. 2.43   Herpes. Cervicitis in a primary attack.

pregnancy (Fig. 2.45), or who have other systemic conditions, e.g. diabetes mellitus, the infection may be more severe and prolonged. Patients often have associated systemic symptoms, including headache, fever, malaise and myalgia. Sacral radiculitis, causing urinary retention, and neurological complications may also occur.

In the primary attack the herpetic lesions shed viral particles for up to 12 days and new lesions may appear in crops until about the 10th day. The lesions crust and healing takes a further 5–10 days.

Some individuals suffer from recurrent episodes of genital herpes; some patients may recognize a prodrome before the vesicles appear. The site of the recurrences depends upon the sensory distribution of the nerve root down which the virus travels. Recurrences vary in presentation from completely asymptomatic episodes of viral shedding to multiple lesions with severe discomfort, but in general they are less severe than the primary attack (Fig. 2.46). Some patients recognize 'trigger factors' that precipitate a recurrence. These include stress, fatigue and vigorous intercourse.

There are other causes of painful genital erosions. Chancroid most closely resembles herpes in its clinical presentation, frequently having multiple erosions. Syphilis should also be excluded. Traumatic genital ulcers, chronic dermatitis and severe candidal infection may also mimic genital herpes. Other viral or erosive diseases should also be considered.

The diagnosis may be confirmed by direct identification of the virus using electron microscopy (Fig. 2.47). The most sensitive technique is virus isolation in tissue culture. Antigen tests are available but these are not as reliable as culture, which remains the method of choice.

Treatment with the antiviral drug acyclovir prevents viral replication. If given orally, 200 mg five times a day for 5 days, acyclovir reduces the length of viral shedding and shortens the healing time in the primary attack. The early application of acyclovir cream may limit recurrences in patients with a prodrome. Suppressive therapy with acyclovir should be considered for a limited period in women suffering from multiple or prolonged recurrences.

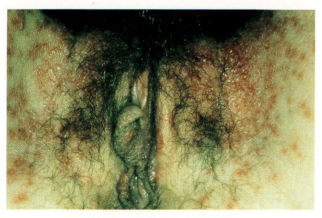

Fig. 2.44 Widespread superficial erosions in a woman with herpes and eczema.

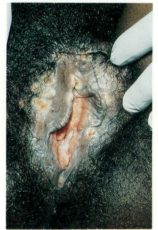

Fig. 2.45 Primary genital herpes in a pregnant woman. Note the multiple large ulcers beginning to scab.

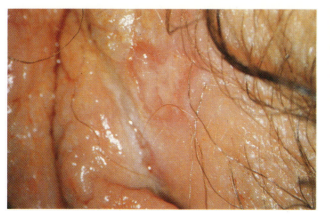

Fig. 2.46 Recurrent herpes. Single irregular ulcer with erythematous halo.

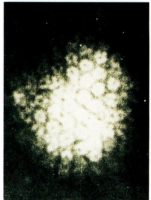

Fig. 2.47 Herpes simplex virus seen under the electron microscope.

HERPES ZOSTER

Herpes zoster, or shingles, is caused by the varicella-zoster virus. The virus remains latent in the ganglia of sensory nerves. Paraesthesia or pain in the dermatome supplied by a sensory nerve is felt before the appearance of skin lesions. Lumbosacral nerves are involved in 15 per cent of cases.

The rash is unilateral and vesicles erupt on an area of erythema, usually in a single dermatome. These rapidly become pustules, which become crusted (Figs 2.48–2.50); occasionally they form bullae and may become haemorrhagic. Inguinal lymphadenopathy often occurs with the eruption, and vaginal lesions have been recorded; there may be associated urinary symptoms. The lesions are usually painful and the pain may persist for months afterwards (post-herpetic neuralgia).

Vulval zoster is usually an easy clinical diagnosis but culture of the vesicle fluid distinguishes it from herpes simplex. Other differential diagnoses include drug eruptions and syphilis.

Specific treatment is not usually indicated. General measures to avoid secondary infection are important. In patients with abnormal cell-mediated immunity the disease may be more severe and often affects multiple dermatomes (Fig. 2.51). Acyclovir in high dose (800 mg five times a day) may help in selected cases.

PAPILLOMA VIRUS INFECTIONS

This heading refers to a wide spectrum of warty

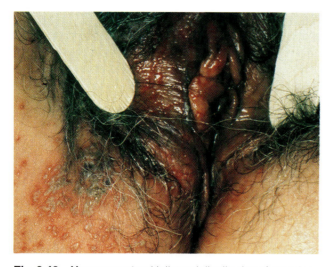

Fig. 2.48   Herpes zoster. Unilateral distribution of pustules that are beginning to crust.

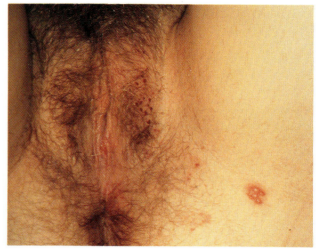

Fig. 2.49   Herpes zoster. Group of pustules seen in the groin with lesions scattered in the pubic hair.

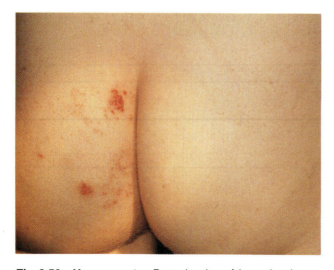

Fig. 2.50   Herpes zoster. Posterior view of the patient in Fig. 2.49. Two distinct areas of pustules with occasional single lesions.

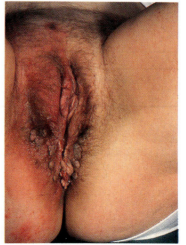

Fig. 2.51   Herpes zoster of the right buttock. Note the co-existence of vaginal warts. The patient was also immunosuppressed.

conditions, indirectly linked to epithelial neoplasia of the vulva and cervix.

The virion of human papilloma virus (HPV) is a spherical particle, 50–55 nm in diameter; the genome is a single molecule of double-stranded DNA (Fig. 2.52). It has not been propagated *in vitro* but molecular virology techniques have shown that there are more than 60 genotypes. Those affecting the vulva are predominantly HPV 6 and 11, usually associated with warts; HPV 16 and 18, usually associated with pre-malignant and malignant epithelial lesions; and occasionally HPV 1–4, which are present in common skin warts.

Genital HPV infections are sexually transmissible; about 60 per cent of current male partners of women with vulval warts have penile warts. Very occasion-ally, warts appear on the genital epithelium through contact with common warts on the hands.

Vulval HPV infection may be manifested as clinical or subclinical lesions or it may be latent, with no discernible disease. The clinical lesions are con-dylomata acuminata (Fig. 2.53) and papular (sessile) warts (Fig. 2.54). Condylomata acuminata commonly affect the fourchette and adjacent labia, but other parts of the vulva, the perineum, anus, vagina and cervix may also be involved (Fig. 2.55). The condylomas are soft, fleshy and vascular and may coalesce into large masses. Papular warts appear on dry areas such as the labia majora; they are usually multiple, raised and 1–3 mm in diameter. Subclinical lesions are visible only if the epithelium is treated with 5% acetic acid and examined with magnification under a bright light. On

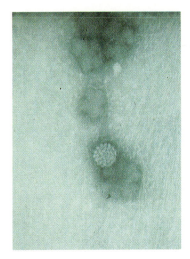

Fig. 2.52   Virus particle from a vulval wart.

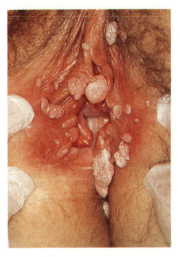

Fig. 2.53   Vulval condylomata acuminata.

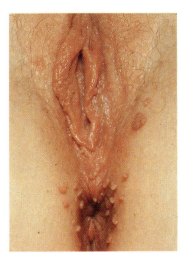

Fig. 2.54   Sessile vulval and peri-anal warts.

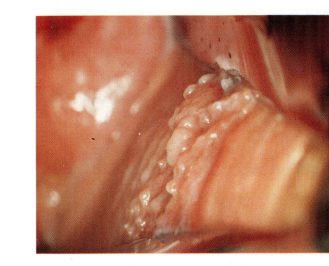

Fig. 2.55   Condylomata acuminata in the vaginal vault.
These are usually associated with vulval warts but they may occur alone.

the vulva, areas of acetowhite epithelium of varied size may appear, particularly on the fourchette. Subclinical HPV infection (Figs 2.56–8) is common on the cervix—'flat condylomas' can be detected colposcopically and there is a characteristic cytology. About 50 per cent of women with vulval warts show evidence of cervical HPV infection, cervical intra-epithelial neoplasia, or both.

Genital warts enlarge if there is impaired immunity, e.g. in patients who are pregnant, suffering from HIV infection or lymphoma or who are immunosuppressed after renal transplant—when the warts may reach a substantial size (Figs 2.59 and 2.60). Giant condyloma is a rare tumour on the vulva—it is large and locally destructive, but does not metastasize and is histologically benign (Fig. 2.61). Its nature is not understood. Malignant change in vulval warts is rare.

The lesions of vulval HPV infection must be distinguished from fibro-epithelial polyps, molluscum contagiosum, the papules and condylomata lata of secon-

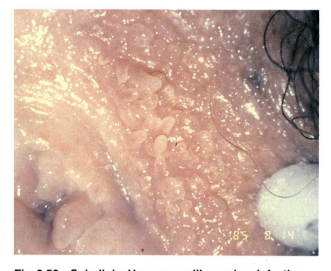

Fig. 2.56   Subclinical human papilloma virus infection. These multiple lesions are too small to be visible without magnification.

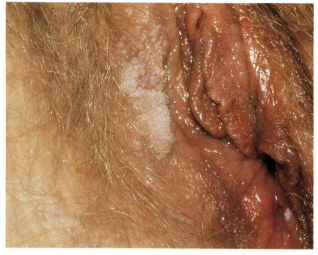

Fig. 2.57   Subclinical human papilloma virus infection. An area of acetowhite epithelium after the application of 5% acetic acid. Histologically, this lesion was a typical wart but 25 per cent of acetowhite genital epithelia show non-specific changes.

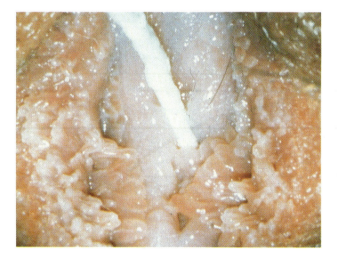

Fig. 2.58   Subclinical human papilloma virus infection. There are extensive acetowhite changes around the introitus. Women with lesions of this sort may complain of superficial dyspareunia.

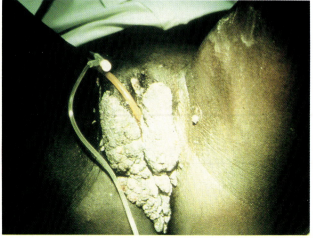

Fig. 2.59   Large condylomata acuminata in pregnancy. Occasionally these may become so large that they obstruct delivery; they regress rapidly in the puerperium.

dary syphilis, benign vulval tumours and from vulval intra-epithelial neoplasia and squamous cell carcinoma.

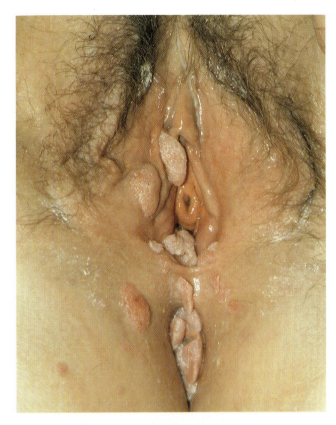

Fig. 2.60 Large indolent condylomata in a patient with defective cell-mediated immunity due to lymphoma. These condylomata respond poorly to treatment, and may progress to vulval intra-epithelial neoplasia.

Biopsy of vulval condylomata is not essential if the clinical appearance is typical, but is essential for atypical lesions. The histology of genital warts shows variable papillomatosis and acanthosis. Koilocytes are large vacuolated cells, often binucleate, present in the outer layers of the lesion; they are pathognomonic of HPV infection (Fig. 2.62).

Associated STD should be excluded and cervical cytology performed on all patients before treatment. Sexual partners should be examined if possible. Applications of 20% podophyllin in spirit once or twice a week are often effective against condylomata acuminata of recent origin. Old keratinized warts and papular warts are best treated by cryotherapy or by cautery or electrodesiccation under local anaesthesia. Subclinical HPV disease of the cervix can be treated by cryotherapy, diathermy or carbon dioxide laser; on the vulva it is probably best left alone.

Anogenital HPV infection in children

Anogenital warts in a child may be caused by:

1. infection from the mother during delivery if she had genital warts;
2. accidental infection within a household through sharing baths and toiletries, or via fomites;
3. infection of the area by HPV from warts on the hands;
4. sexual abuse.

In female children both condylomata acuminata and sessile warts may appear around the vulva or anus; the former may reach a substantial size, and become

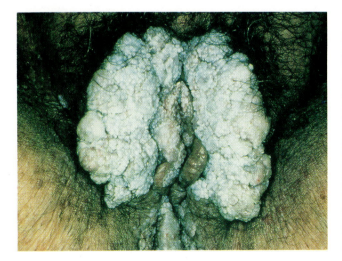

Fig. 2.61 Giant condyloma. Although these large tumours are locally destructive, they do not metastasize and are histologically benign, being composed of condyloma acuminatum tissue.

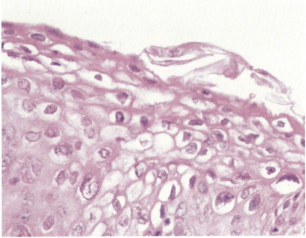

Fig. 2.62 Histology of a vulval wart, showing acanthosis and numerous vacuolated koilocytes.

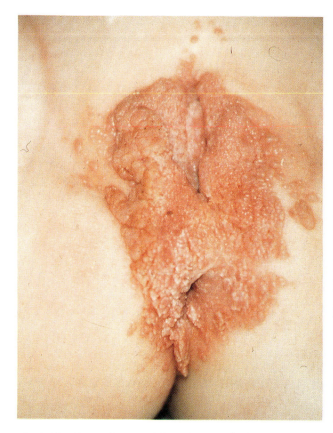

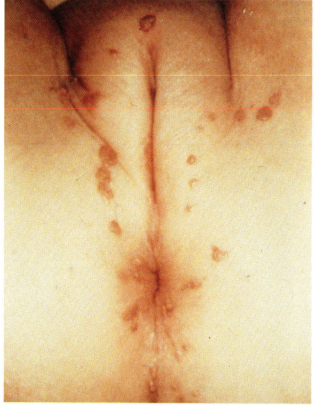

Fig. 2.63 Extensive condylomata acuminata surrounding the vulva in an infant.

Fig. 2.64 Multiple sessile peri-anal and perivulval warts in a young child. The possibility of sexual abuse must be considered in all cases of anogenital warts in children.

secondarily infected (Figs 2.63 and 2.64).

A child with anogenital warts may have been sexually assaulted and, in view of the medicolegal implications, thorough investigation is essential. Biopsy should be performed if there is the slightest doubt about the diagnosis and associated STD should be excluded by appropriate laboratory tests. There may be no clinical features to indicate the actual source of the warts (see Chapter 7). Enquiry should be made about a history of genital warts in the child's mother or other family members. It is possible to establish the genotype present in anogenital warts by molecular virology, but the clinical, epidemiological or medicolegal value of this procedure has not yet been decided.

MOLLUSCUM CONTAGIOSUM

Molluscum contagiosum (MC) is a benign papular dermatosis that is often sexually transmitted.

The virus of MC is a poxvirus (Fig. 2.65). It replicates in the cytoplasm of infected cells where it forms large inclusions; eventually the nucleus disappears and the cell is entirely occupied by virus—the 'molluscum contagiosum body' (Fig. 2.66). The virus has never been replicated *in vitro*.

The incubation period is 2–6 weeks. In children lesions appear on the face, trunk and limbs but in adults, when they appear on the genitals, MC is a sexually transmitted disease (Fig. 2.67). In women, MC affects the lower abdomen, pubis, labia majors and adjacent skin. The smallest lesions are rounded pink–grey papules but as they enlarge they become umbilicated and 2–5 mm in diameter (Fig. 2.68). Between 1 and 20 lesions are usually present but they become larger and more numerous in people who are immunosuppressed. Histologically, an MC lesion shows acanthosis, with a central core of MC bodies and cell debris.

The lesions of MC may be mistaken for warts or may resemble other papular vulval conditions, such as basal cell carcinoma, but their umbilicated appearance is characteristic. For laboratory diagnosis the core of the lesion may be scraped out and examined as a wet preparation for MC bodies, or biopsy may be performed.

The lesions can be destroyed by liquid phenol introduced on a pointed stick, curetted under local anaesthesia or treated by cryotherapy.

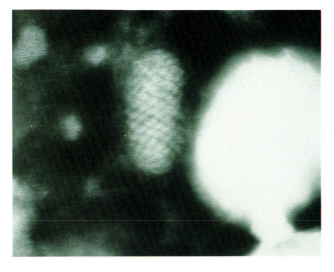

Fig. 2.65   Virus particle from a molluscum contagiosum lesion.

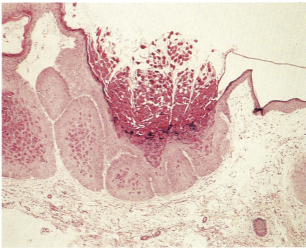

Fig. 2.66   Histology of a molluscum contagiosum lesion. There is acanthosis and the central core is filled with molluscum contagiosum bodies and cell debris.

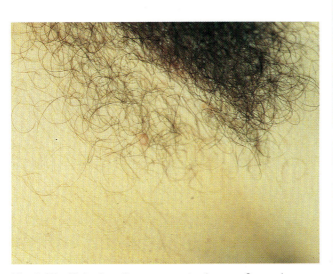

Fig. 2.67   Vulval molluscum contagiosum. Several umbilicated papules are visible.

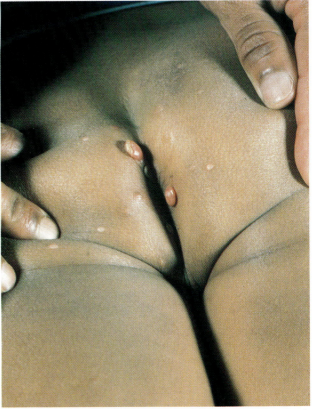

Fig. 2.68   Large peri-anal molluscum contagiosum lesions in a child.

3. Non-infective, Non-neoplastic Conditions

VULVAL MANIFESTATIONS OF SYSTEMIC DISEASES

Vulval manifestations of systemic disease are uncommon:

Acrodermatitis enteropathica

Acrodermatitis enteropathica is referred to on page 88.

Glucagonoma syndrome

Glucagonoma is a rare pancreatic tumour, resulting in diabetes, stomatitis, weight loss and a striking circinate erythematous and bullous rash, necrolytic migratory erythema, in the genital area and elsewhere (Fig. 3.1).

Inflammatory bowel disease

Crohn's disease is more commonly associated with anogenital lesions than is ulcerative colitis (Figs 3.2 and 3.3). Lesions may antedate the onset or detection of bowel disease and need not be anatomically continuous with the bowel. Sinuses and ulcers, fistulae and abscesses mingle with inflamed peri-anal tags and oedema. The oedema may be unilateral or generalized, and in extreme cases results in vulval lymphangiectasia (Fig. 3.4). Granulomatous cheilitis or changes

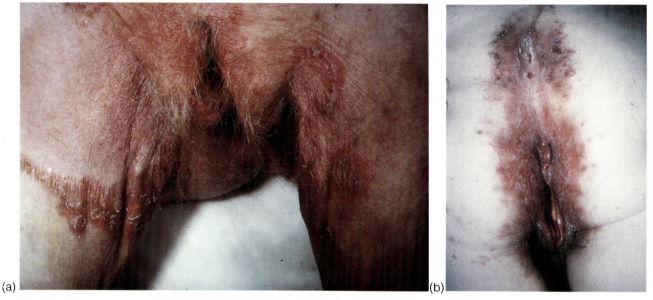

(a) (b)

Fig. 3.1 Glucagonoma. (a) Circinate erythematous and (b) bullous eruption of anogenital area.

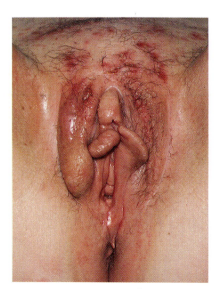

**Fig. 3.2
Crohn's disease.**
Marked firm
induration and
swelling.

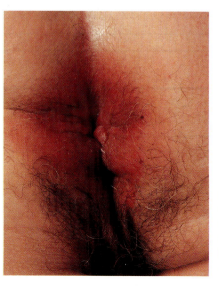

**Fig. 3.3
Crohn's disease.**
Redness, induration and tag-like
lesions perianally.

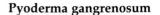

in the oral mucosa referred to as cobblestone-like are often present. Management of the bowel disease (e.g. by metronidazole) can improve the skin lesions. Local symptomatic measures and minor surgical intervention are also beneficial.

Diabetes

Erythrasma is quite common in diabetics (Fig. 3.5), particularly in black patients, and candidosis is extremely common in newly diagnosed or uncontrolled diabetics (Fig. 3.6). It is probable that pruritus vulvae in diabetics is always related to *Candida* infection.

Pyoderma gangrenosum

This condition may occasionally affect the vulva. It is strongly associated with rheumatoid arthritis and ulcerative colitis but may occur in the apparent absence of an underlying pathology (Fig. 3.7). The ulcers are indolent, with a dusky overhanging edge, and are sometimes grouped as small 'pepper-pot' lesions. Histology may be non-specific or may show a vasculitis.

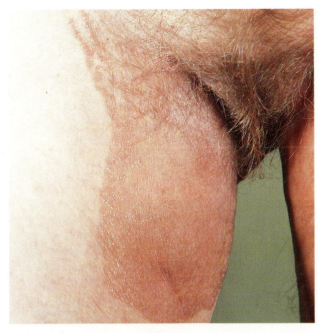

Fig. 3.5   Erythrasma in a diabetic. Brown, finely-scaling lesions.

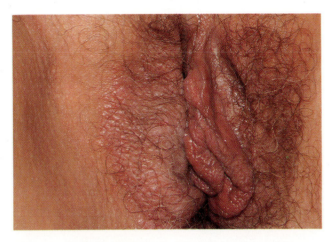

Fig. 3.4   Crohn's disease. Swelling and erythema with lymphangiectasia.

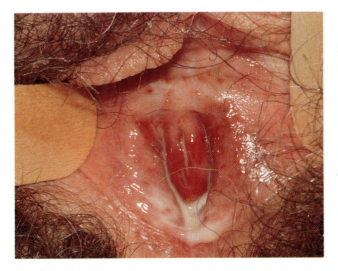

Fig. 3.6   Candidosis in an uncontrolled diabetic. Note the redness and the thick discharge. This patient also had herpes simplex virus infection.

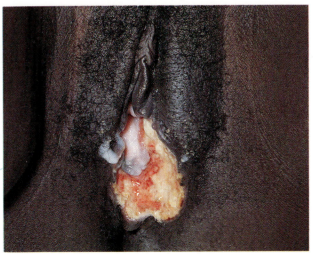

Fig. 3.7   A deep acute vulval ulcer with an overhanging edge in an otherwise healthy woman of 28. The histology showed an acute necrotizing vasculitis and the lesion healed rapidly with oral prednisolone. The most likely diagnosis was pyoderma gangrenosum.

It is important to differentiate pyoderma gangrenosum from infective lesions, and especially from synergistic bacterial gangrene, which has a predilection for the vulva and which responds to débridement and antibiotics. Systemic steroids and dapsone and minocycline are indicated in pyoderma gangrenosum.

Behçet's syndrome

The oculo-orogenital form of this multisystem disease may affect the vulva (Fig. 3.8). The ulcers are painful, shallow, single or multiple and usually on the labia minora; they usually, but not always, result in scarring. Colchicine and systemic steroids are of benefit and the topical application of a corticosteroid, particularly in the form of a combination of triamcinolone with tetracycline, can also help.

VULVAL ULCERS

Vulval ulcers without evidence of Behçet's syndrome are usually painful and recurrent (Fig. 3.9) and of the aphthous variety. Various clinical patterns of uncertain significance have been described; oral ulceration is often associated (Fig. 3.10). A triamcinolone/tetracycline combination applied topically is helpful.

GENETIC DISORDERS

Many rare conditions affect the vulva and will usually show lesions elsewhere. An example is the white sponge naevus associated with oral lesions (Fig. 3.11); another is Darier's disease in which the typical brownish keratotic papules are common in the genital area and frequently become secondarily infected. See also Hailey-Hailey disease, p. 44.

DISORDERS OF THE HAIR

Alopecia areata

Alopecia areata—where there is patchy or complete loss of hair with no scarring or inflammation—occasionally affects the hair of the genital region (Fig. 3.12).

Folliculitis

Inflammatory papules and boils may affect the mons pubis and peri-anal area.

Pilonidal sinuses

Sinuses containing hairs are found occasionally.

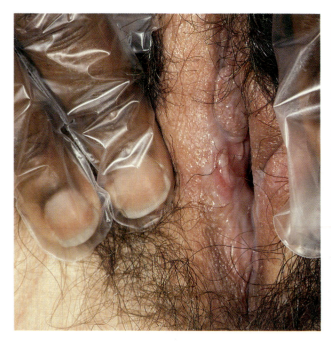

Fig. 3.8 Behçet's syndrome. Ulceration of the vulva.

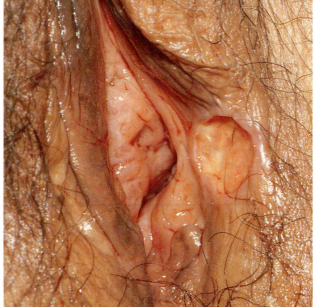

Fig. 3.9 Recurrent painful vulval ulcers, aphthous in type. Such patients are often categorized as having Behçet's disease without supporting evidence. This patient had had oral ulcers since childhood and two siblings were similarly affected.

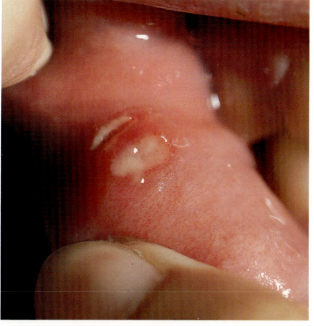

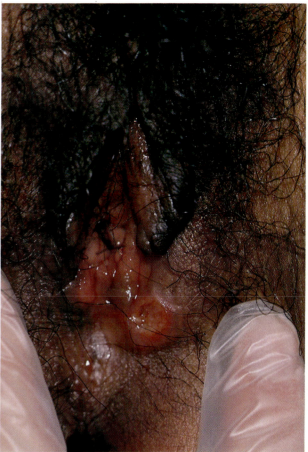

Fig. 3.10   Aphthous ulcers. (a) Lesions of the mouth.
(b) Lesions of the vulva.

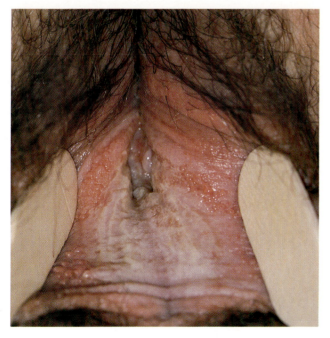

Fig. 3.11   White sponge naevus of mouth and vulva.
There was a family history of this rare condition.

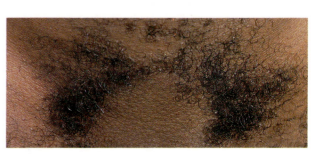

**Fig. 3.12   Alopecia areata showing smooth
non-inflamed alopecia of the mons pubis.** Lesions may or
may not be present elsewhere.

DISORDERS OF PIGMENTATION

Pigmented lesions

Pigmented lesions may be related to melanin or haemosiderin.

Melanin-related lesions include pigmented neo-plasms (vulval intra-epithelial neoplasia (VIN) (Fig. 3.13), basal cell carcinoma (Fig. 3.14), moles and melanoma, lentigo and melanosis) and postinflammatory pigmentation, particularly in a dark skin and in relation to lichen planus (Fig. 3.15). Acanthosis nigricans (Fig. 3.16) is a very rare cause of marked hyperpigmentation. Pseudo-acanthosis nigricans

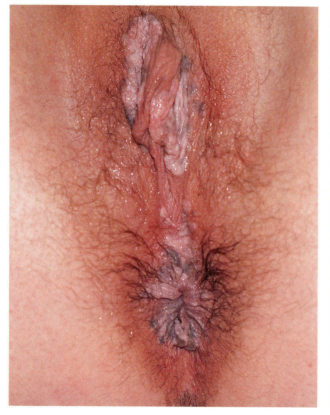

Fig. 3.13 Pigmented vulval intra-epithelial neoplasia.

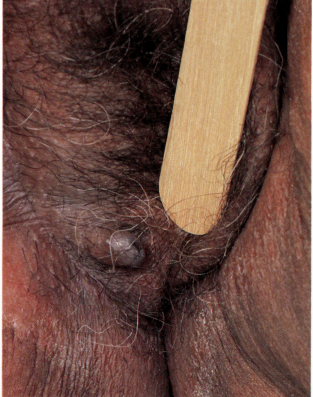

Fig. 3.14 Pigmented basal cell carcinoma.

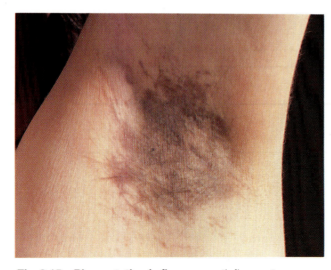

Fig. 3.15 Pigmentation in flexure, postinflammatory following lichen planus.

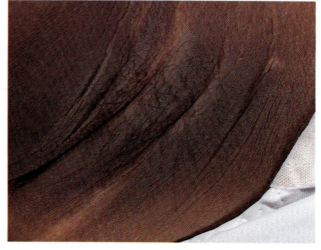

Fig. 3.16 Acanthosis nigricans. Papillomatosis and pigmentation in flexures.

(Fig. 3.17) is relatively common in dark-skinned obese patients, the pigmentation often being accompanied by skin tags.

Haemosiderin, a brownish-red iron–protein compound, is often found in lichen sclerosus, in some cases of vestibulitis and in caruncles (Fig. 3.18).

Hypopigmentation

Hypopigmentation is a feature of lichen sclerosus (Fig. 3.19). Postinflammatory hypopigmentation is seen in dark skins. The total depigmentation of vitiligo may affect the vulval area, where it is usually striking and symmetrical (Figs 3.20 and 3.21).

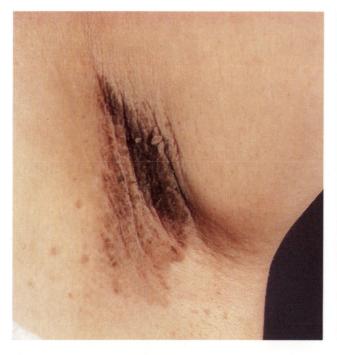

Fig. 3.17 Pseudo-acanthosis nigricans. Darkening of a flexure with tags in an obese individual. These changes will regress if weight is lost.

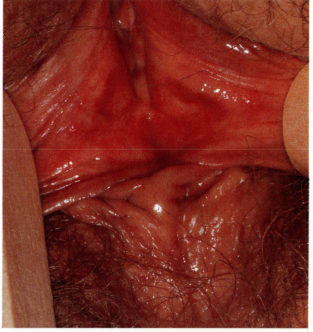

Fig. 3.18 Deposition of haemosiderin in vestibulitis.

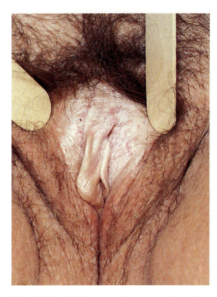

Fig. 3.19 Lichen sclerosus. Note the striking pallor.

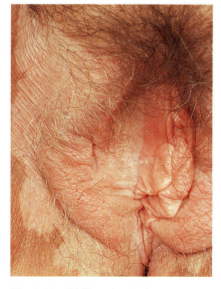

Fig. 3.20 Vitiligo. Loss of pigmentation, without inflammation or change of texture.

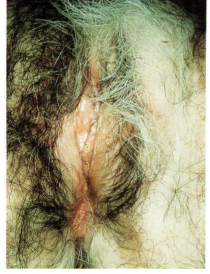

Fig. 3.21 Vitiligo. The hair is often white in the affected area.

SEBACEOUS GLANDS

Yellowish punctate or confluent lesions are not uncommon between the labia and on the inner aspects of the labia minora; they are a variant of normal (Fordyce condition) (Fig. 3.22). Sebaceous material tends to form papules, nodules and cysts, which may be multiple and persistent; simple surgical measures are effective in such cases.

APOCRINE GLANDS

Fox–Fordyce disease

Fox–Fordyce disease is an inflammatory condition of the apocrine glands. Closely-set itching papules are scattered over the vulva and pubic area and are often found at other sites of apocrine activity, e.g. the breast (Fig. 3.23) and axillae. The symptoms regress after the menopause. The intense itching can be helped to some extent by topical corticosteroids or retinoic acid, or by the oral contraceptive.

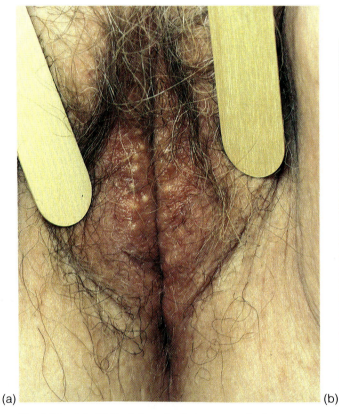

(a)

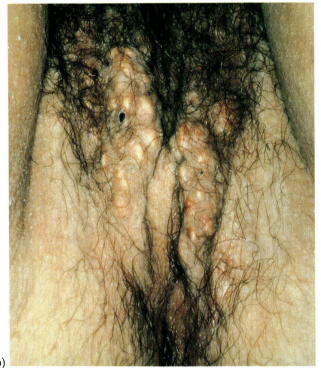

(b)

Fig. 3.22   (a), (b) Nodules of sebaceous material.

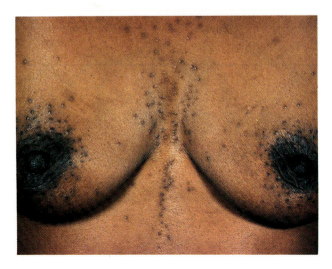

Fig. 3.23   Fox–Fordyce disease. Multiple papules at the site of apocrine gland activity, here on the breasts. The papules give rise to cyclical pruritus.

Hidradenitis suppurativa

Hidradenitis suppurativa also affects the apocrine glands but is much more common than Fox–Fordyce disease. Starting after puberty, it occurs in the anogenital area, particularly in the groin but also in the axillae and on the breasts. Milder cases show recurrent inflammatory lesions with painful swellings and abscesses leading to bridged scars with comedones (Fig. 3.24). In severe cases there is widespread swelling and destruction of tissue with sinuses. The aetiology is probably related to androgen metabolism and treatment is often with a combination of anti-androgens and antibiotics. In severe cases surgery is probably the best answer. Neoplasia has been reported as a rare complication.

BULLOUS DERMATOSES

Some blistering eruptions have a predilection for the vulva.

Stevens–Johnson syndrome

Stevens–Johnson syndrome is a form of erythema multiforme with mucosal involvement; it may be related to drugs or to infection, notably herpes simplex virus, although idiopathic cases may occur (Fig. 3.25). Ulceration following upon the bullae may be discrete or confluent. Oral and/or ocular lesions are often present with or without skin involvement (Fig. 3.26). Symptomatic treatment is indicated and systemic steroids are contra-indicated. Toxic epidermal nec-

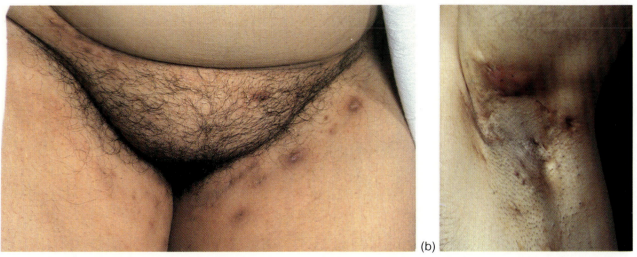

(a)   (b)

Fig. 3.24 Hidradenitis suppurativa. (a) Extensive scarring in the groins. **(b)** Bridged scarring and comedones in the axilla.

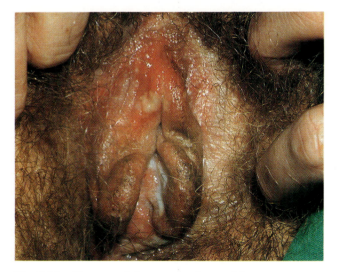

Fig. 3.25 Stevens–Johnson syndrome. Ulcers are consequent upon bullae in this form of erythema multiforme with mucosal involvement.

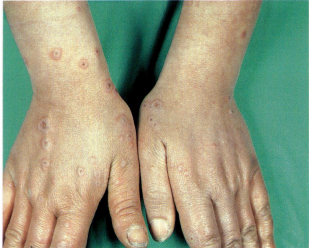

Fig. 3.26 'Target' or 'iris' lesions of erythema multiforme **on the hands.**

41

rolysis must be considered in the differential diagnosis, although it is probably true to say that there is some overlap between the two conditions.

Pemphigus vulgaris and cicatricial pemphigoid

Pemphigoid which is an immunobullous disease rarely affects the vulva; pemphigus vulgaris and cicatricial pemphigoid however, also immunobullous conditions, are often located at the vulva. Direct im-

munofluorescence shows immunoglobulins at various sites (Fig. 3.27 a and b).

Pemphigus vulgaris
Pemphigus vulgaris is a rare condition with a predilection for the Jewish race. Other lesions—mucosal or cutaneous—are usual but not invariable. Bullae are often confluent and erode to form painful raw areas; lesions may extend into the vagina (Fig. 3.28). There is no scarring.

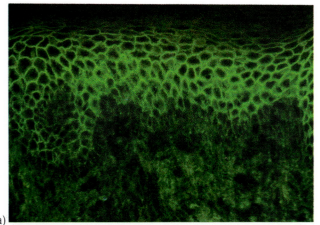
(a)

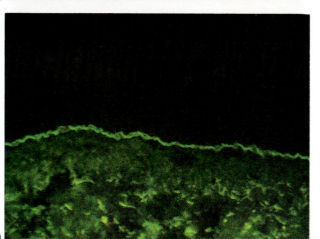
(b)

Fig. 3.27 Direct immunofluorescence. (a) A patient with pemphigus showing intercellular IgG. **(b)** Immunoglobulin usually IgG deposited at the basement membrane zone as is found in cicatricial pemphigoid.

Fig. 3.28 Pemphigus. Confluent moist erythema and massed, superficial, easily ruptured bullae. The patient had extensive lesions of the trunk and oropharynx.

The histology, which shows intra-epidermal bullae with acantholysis, and the direct and indirect immunofluorescence findings (Fig. 3.27), which demonstrate antibodies directed against the intercellular substance of the epidermis, are diagnostic and essential, as treatment is long-term and not free from side-effects. High-dose oral steroids and other immunosuppressive agents are required.

Cicatricial pemphigoid

Cicatricial pemphigoid often shows vulval manifestations and lesions on other areas may or may not be present (Figs 3.29–3.33). Scarring is a feature and its consequences may be serious if it involves the vagina, the eyes and the oropharynx. Histological examination, which should always be carried out, will demon-

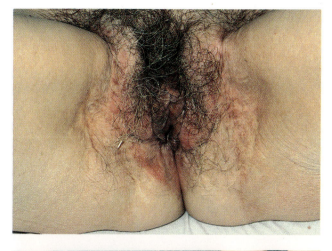

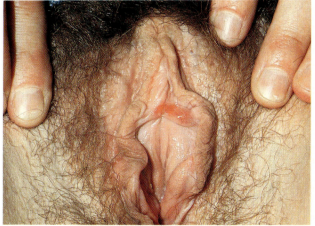

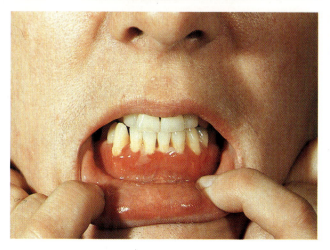

Fig. 3.29 Cicatricial pemphigoid. Extensive scarring following bullae at the vulva.

Fig. 3.30 Cicatricial pemphigoid. A localized eroded area.

Fig. 3.31 Cicatricial pemphigoid. Desquamative inflammatory gingivitis (which also has other causes, e.g. pemphigus, lichen planus).

strate a subepidermal bulla; direct immunofluorescence will usually demonstrate immunoglobulin at the basement membrane zone and occasionally circulating antibodies are to be found. Topical corticosteroids will help mild lesions but the patient will usually need oral steroids or dapsone.

Familial benign chronic pemphigus (Hailey–Hailey disease)

This condition is inherited as an autosomal dominant characteristic. Lesions affect the anogenital area and other flexures. They are often precipitated or worsened by contact allergy or infection. They are moist, scaly and erythematous, and hence easily mistaken for eczematous conditions (Fig. 3.34). Histology, which is diagnostic, showing extensive acantholysis, should always be checked if progress of such lesions is unusually slow or if there are suspicious features. Immunofluorescence is negative. Treatment with topical corticosteroids and topical and oral anti-infective agents is usually satisfactory but oral steroids are occasionally required. Possible contact factors should be explored.

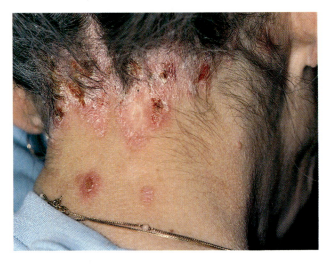

Fig. 3.32 Cicatricial pemphigoid. Scarring and milia formation on the neck.

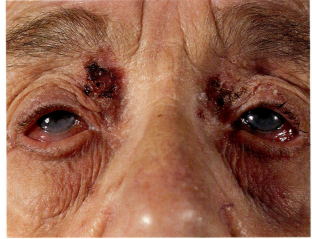

Fig. 3.33 Cicatricial pemphigoid. Typical obliteration of conjunctival sulci.

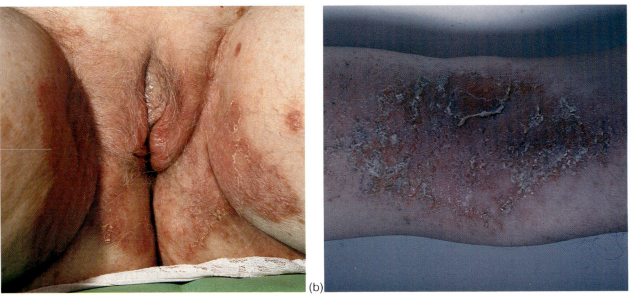

(a) (b)

Fig. 3.34 Familial benign chronic pemphigus. (a) Moist fissured erythematous plaques extending into the genitocrural folds. These lesions were dramatically worsened by infection. **(b)** Typical morphology at an extragenital site: note moist fissuring.

Intertrigo

Intertrigo is a common inflammatory condition of flexures, facilitated by obesity, heat and sweating (Fig. 3.35). It readily becomes secondarily infected and when *Candida* is present small satellite lesions appear. Treatment depends largely on dealing with predisposing factors; separation of folds is important.

Psoriasis

The psoriatic diathesis is genetically determined. Lesions in flexures are quite common and are usually but not invariably accompanied by lesions elsewhere (Figs 3.36 and 3.37). The local environment is responsible for the relative absence of the typical parakeratotic scale. Management is by bland emollients and mild corticosteroids.

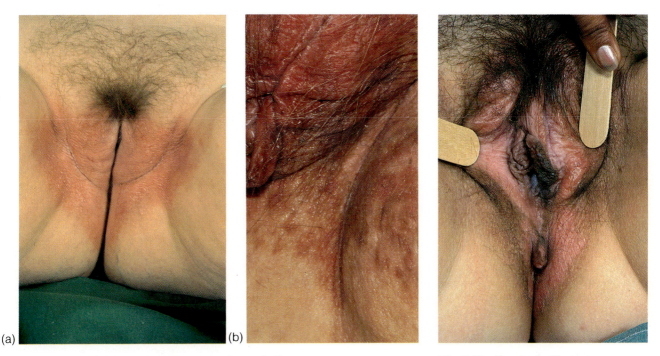

(a)   (b)

Fig. 3.35 (a) Diffuse intertriginous erythema in the genitocrural folds. (b) Candida in diabetes.

Fig. 3.36 Psoriasis. The lesions are less scaly than those elsewhere but the well-defined edge and bright erythema are typical.

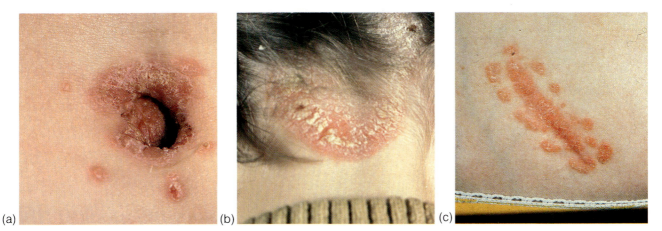

(a)   (b)   (c)

Fig. 3.37 Typical lesions of psoriasis. (a) At umbilicus. **(b)** At the back of the neck. **(c)** As the Koebner phenomenon in an appendicectomy scar.

ECZEMA

Eczema is characterized by spongiosis, acanthosis and a perivascular, mainly lymphocytic, dermal infiltrate. Its causes are various and it may be considered as synonymous with dermatitis. On occasion, the eczema appears to be idiopathic.

Although the vulva is often spared in severe atopic dermatitis, eczematous vulval lesions are sometimes apparent in the absence of involvement elsewhere in patients with an atopic background. The affected area is red, scaly and often moist. Lichenification (thickening caused by rubbing and scratching) is marked (Figs 3.38–3.40).

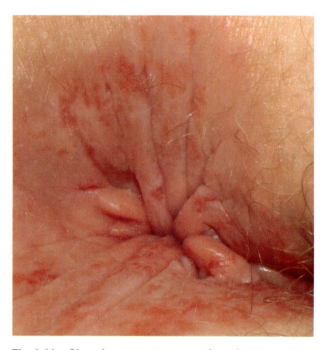

Fig. 3.38 Chronic eczematous eruption of vulva and peri-anal area. Note the lichenification round the anal orifice.

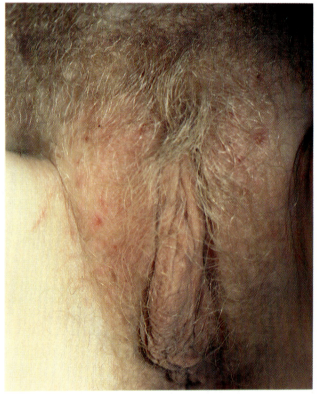

Fig. 3.39 Eczema. General erythema and lichenification.

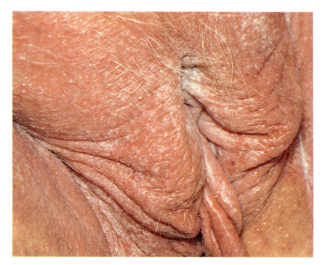

Fig. 3.40 Eczema. Marked lichenification.

Seborrhoeic dermatitis may also affect the vulva. The lesions are diffusely red and the natal cleft area is often affected (Fig. 3.41).

It is often difficult to distinguish between these forms of eczema and identification will usually depend on the history and on the study of lesions elsewhere. Management of acute severe cases is by bathing with saline or potassium permanganate diluted to 1 in 10 000, followed by the application of a corticosteroid cream. Bland emollients and corticosteroid preparations are effective later in the course of treatment. Treatment for secondary infection is often necessary. Superimposed contact dermatitis from topical applications is often relevant and is investigated by patch testing, a specialized procedure best carried out by the dermatologist (Figs 3.42 and 3.43).

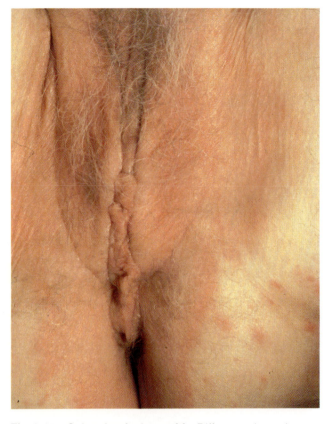

Fig. 3.41 Seborrhoeic dermatitis. Diffuse erythema in a patient with seborrhoeic dermatitis at the vulva.

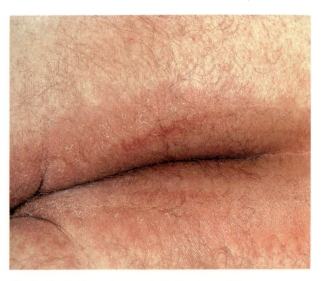

Fig. 3.42 Peri-anal rash related to dermatitis medicamentosa (allergy to ointment for 'piles' containing a local anaesthetic). Such lesions occur at the vulva following the use of similar applications for pruritus, as well as with antiseptic or antibiotic preparations. The diagnosis is confirmed by patch testing.

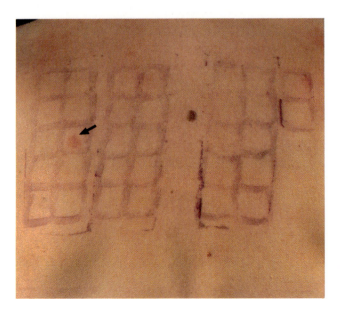

Fig. 3.43 Patch tests on the back at the second reading showing a strong positive reaction to neomycin. Patch tests are applied for 48 h, removed, read immediately and then read again after a further few days.

LICHEN SIMPLEX

'Lichen simplex' is the term given to lichenification (thickening) brought about by itching and subsequent rubbing of apparently normal skin (Figs 3.44–3.46). The thickening will resolve with a potent corticosteroid but tends to recur, and it is always important to establish on resolution that the skin is indeed normal because lichenification of, for example, eczema and lichen sclerosus is common. The whole of the vulva may be affected but the labia majora show the most striking changes. They become thickened with accentuation of skin markings; there is pallor related to maceration of the hyperkeratosis.

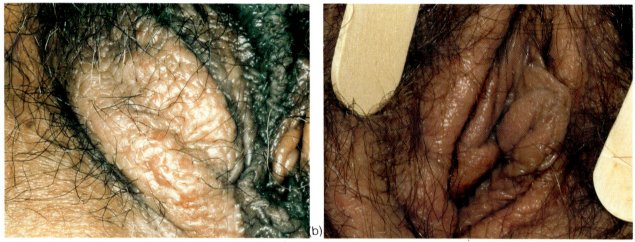

(a)   (b)

Fig. 3.44   **Lichen simplex. Gross thickening of labia majora.** Pale reddish or earthy colouration; no underlying skin lesion.

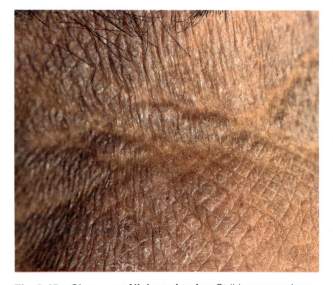

Fig. 3.45   **Close-up of lichen simplex.** Striking example on the neck, another common site for this change.

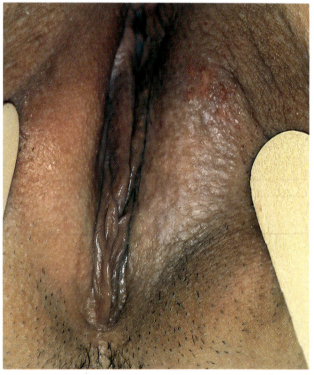

Fig. 3.46   **Lichen simplex.** Where changes are so localized and asymmetrical it is particularly important to exclude such conditions as extramammary Paget's disease.

LICHEN PLANUS

Lichen planus, an idiopathic (possibly auto-immune) dermatosis, affects keratinized skin in the anogenital area. The typical purplish, flat-topped papules are often followed by hyperpigmentation. The lesions are usually easy to recognize and biopsy is rarely necessary. Pruritus is responsive to topical corticosteroids.

Histology will show a characteristic picture with a prominent granular layer and a dense subepidermal band of inflammatory cells coming right up to the basal layer and often resulting in basal cell liquefaction (Fig. 3.47).

There will often be lesions elsewhere on the skin or in the mouth (Figs 3.48–3.52).

Fig. 3.47   Lichen planus. Hyperkeratosis and acanthosis. A prominent granular layer and a dense subepidermal band of inflammatory cells extending up to the basal layer.

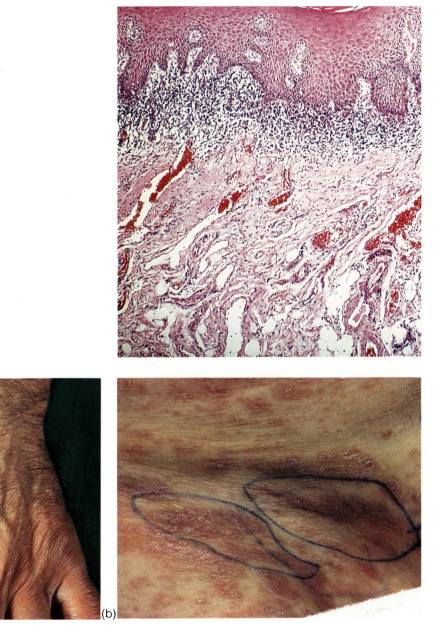

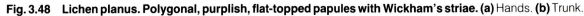

(a)   (b)

Fig. 3.48   Lichen planus. Polygonal, purplish, flat-topped papules with Wickham's striae. (a) Hands. **(b)** Trunk.

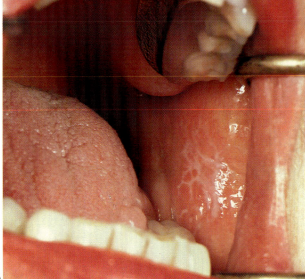

(a)

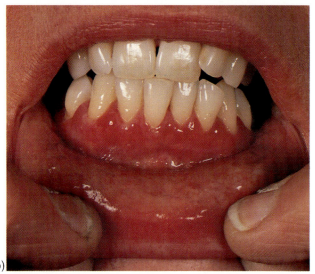

(b)

Fig. 3.49   Lichen planus in the mouth. (a) Typical bluish-white network. **(b)** Erosive gingivitis.

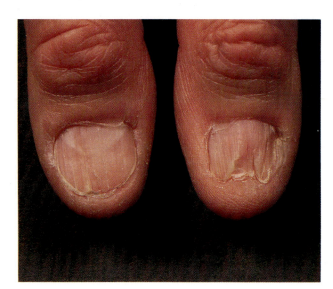

Fig. 3.50   Gross destructive changes of the nails, typical of lichen planus.

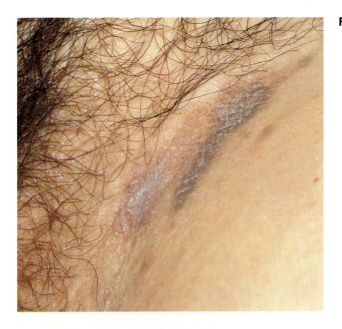

Fig. 3.51   Lichen planus, purplish colour.

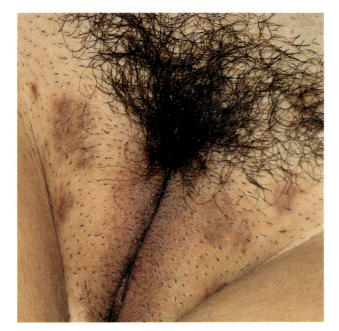

Fig. 3.52   Lichen planus, brownish on resolution.

Erosive lichen planus

An erosive form of lichen planus is also recognized, affecting the inner aspects of the vulva and the vagina (Figs 3.53 and 3.54). The vagina is friable and telangiectatic and often develops adhesions and stenosis. Oral lesions, often erosive, are common in this type, which may or may not be accompanied by lesions on the rest of the skin. Histology in these cases is often non-specific. The differential diagnosis is from eroded vulval intra-epithelial neoplasia and vestibulitis, as well as from other eroded atrophic conditions, e.g. lichen sclerosus and cicatricial pemphigoid. Treatment is unsatisfactory. Topical potent corticosteroids and systemic steroids offer the most help at present, though topical cyclosporin has been reported to be beneficial. It is usually advisable to avoid surgical measures, although minor procedures with scrupulous attention to follow-up and employment of dilators and potent corticosteroids can occasionally be helpful.

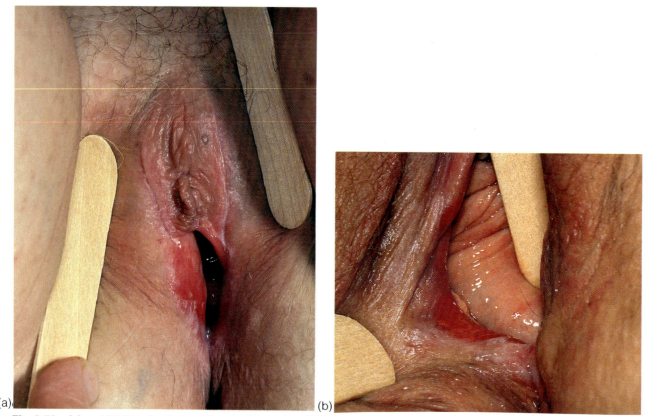

(a)   (b)

Fig. 3.53   (a) and (b) Erosive lichen planus of the vulva. Fiery eroded erythema.

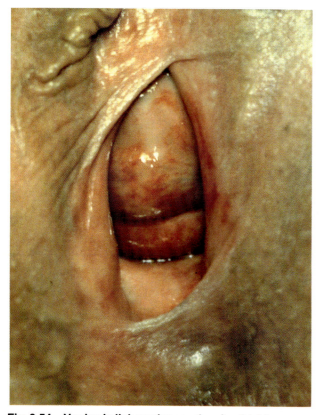

Fig. 3.54   Vagina in lichen planus, showing friable erythema and telangiectasia.

LICHEN SCLEROSUS

Lichen sclerosus was originally described as a variant of lichen planus and the two have many features in common; it has a significant association with auto-immune disease. Although it affects all areas of the body in both sexes (Fig. 3.55), the predilection of lichen sclerosus for the anogenital area in women and girls has led in the past to the erroneous view that anogenital lichen sclerosus was something peculiar to that area and it was not recognized by gynaecologists in particular to have manifestations elsewhere. Consequently the terminology of vulval lesions was for long very confused. This problem is now largely resolved (see Appendix A).

The histological finding of a thinned epidermis with subepidermal hyalinization in which blood vessels are unsupported, and a deeper band of inflammatory cells (Fig. 3.56), explains the clinical findings of atrophy, telangiectasia and purpura.

There is often a figure-of-eight pattern involving the

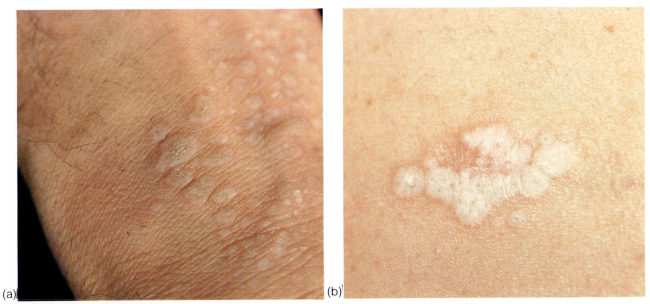

Fig. 3.55   Lichen sclerosus. Typical ivory white papules. **(a)** On the wrist. **(b)** On the trunk.

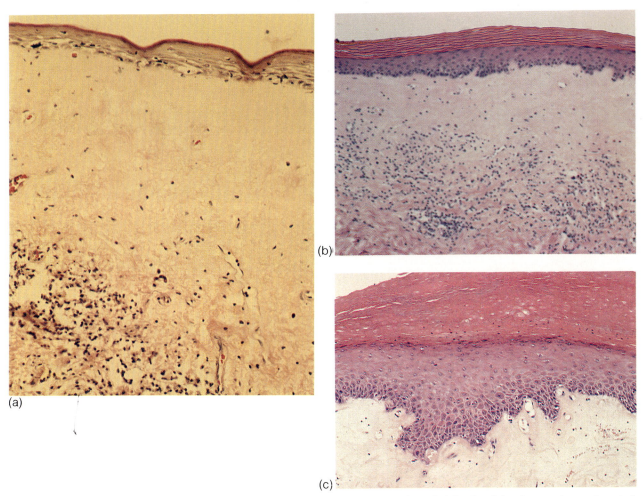

Fig. 3.56   Lichen sclerosus, histological findings. (a) Showing thin epidermis underlying hyalinized zone, deeper band of inflammatory cells. **(b)** and **(c)** Showing some hyperkeratosis, acanthosis, with irregularity of the rete pegs; developments often noted in chronic lichen sclerosus which has been rubbed in response to itching.

vulva and peri-anal area. The most frequently affected parts are the peri-anal area, the genitocrural folds, the inner aspects of the labia majora, all aspects of the labia minora and the tissue round the clitoris (Figs 3.57–3.75). The clitoris is quite often sealed off completely under the preputial folds. Atrophy is usually marked with obliteration of contours. Pallor is striking, often with an added purpuric component. The lesions will readily thicken (lichenification) and can become grossly hyperkeratotic. Thick brittle hyperkeratotic plaques tend to fissure. Fusion in the midline is common and may be extreme. Both signs and symptoms are very variable in this condition. The degree of risk of malignancy is difficult to quantify but almost certainly it is increased in patients with lichen sclerosus who should therefore be kept under supervision. Unfortu-

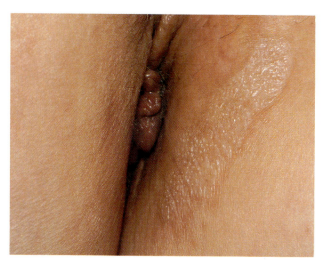

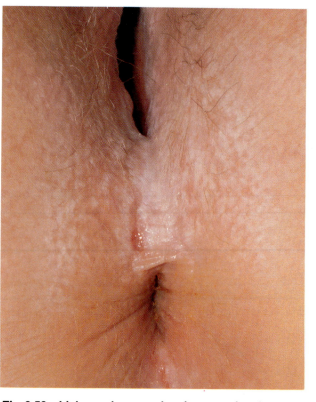

Fig. 3.57   Plaque of lichen sclerosus near the anus.

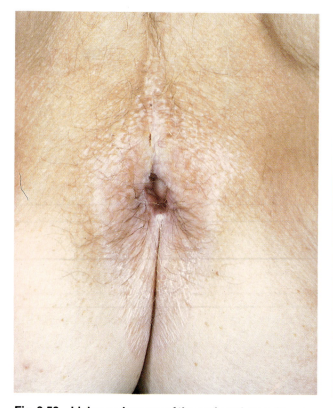

Fig. 3.58   Lichen sclerosus of the peri-anal area. Showing pallor and peripheral papules and typical figure-of-eight pattern.

Fig. 3.59   Lichen sclerosus showing some involvement of the perineum, which is pale, with typical peripheral lichen sclerosus papules. Note the tendency to fissure.

nately, malignancy sometimes supervenes on symptomless lichen sclerosus. Unless malignancy has developed, surgery has no place in management, except occasionally to free fused tissue or to enlarge a stenosed introitus by some form of perineoplasty. Management with bland emollients and, initially, potent topical corticosteroids, which can then be phased out or for which milder ones can be substituted, is usually extremely satisfactory. Topical testosterone has varying success but is not widely used in the UK. Oral retinoids are probably not helpful and are accompanied by serious side-effects.

Lesions in children are described elsewhere (see p. 90).

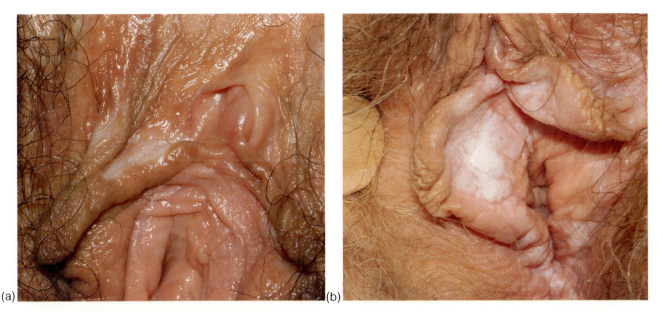

(a) (b)

Fig. 3.60 Minimal lesions of lichen sclerosus. Small areas of whiteness.

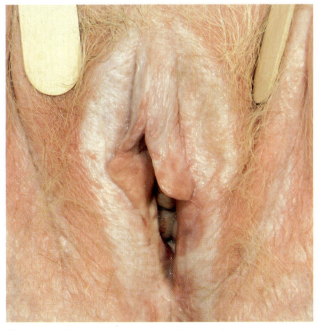

Fig. 3.61 Lichen sclerosus. In this case the appearance is of striking pallor rather than loss of tissue.

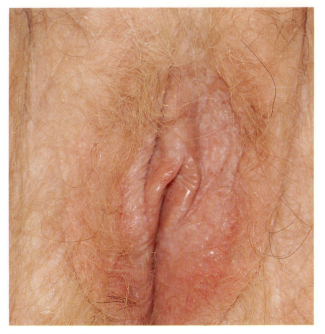

Fig. 3.62 Lichen sclerosus plus vitiligo. The central reddened area is affected by lichen sclerosus, the surrounding white areas are those of vitiligo. Lichen sclerosus is significantly associated with vitiligo.

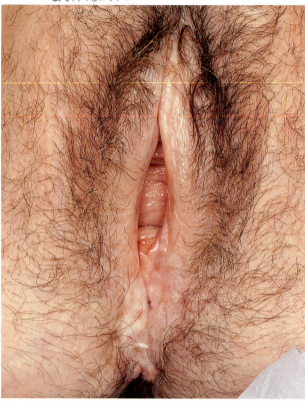

Fig. 3.63 Fusion in lichen sclerosus. In this case of tissue round the clitoris.

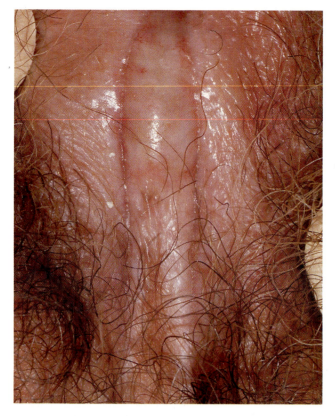

Fig. 3.64 Fusion in lichen sclerosus. More extensive fusion.

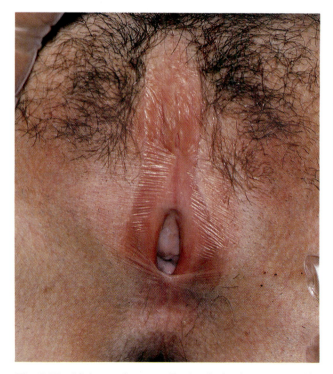

Fig. 3.65 Lichen sclerosus. Further fusion has occurred in this patient.

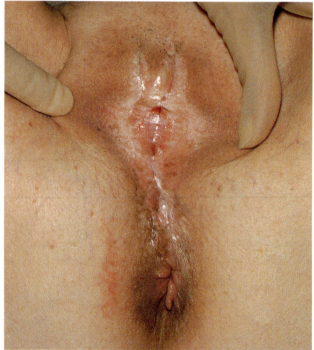

Fig. 3.66 Fusion in lichen sclerosus. Almost complete fusion.

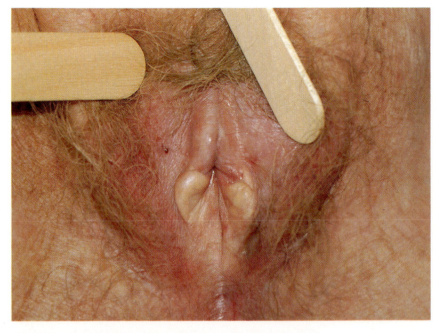

Fig. 3.67   A typically waxy appearance with telangiectasia.

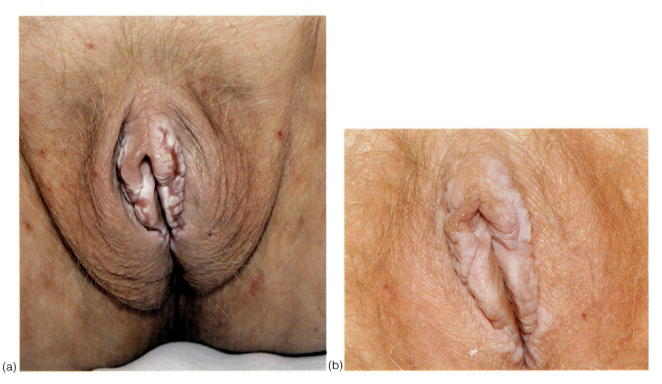

(a)

(b)

Fig. 3.68   Hyperkeratosis and lichenification in lichen sclerosus. (a) and **(b)** Before and after a short period of treatment with a potent corticosteroid.

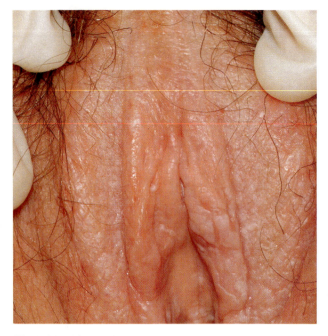

Fig. 3.69   Lichenification of lichen sclerosus in response to rubbing. This would be difficult to differentiate from simple lichenification without biopsy and/or assessment on resolution, but the peripheral rather hyperkeratotic pallor is suggestive of lichen sclerosus.

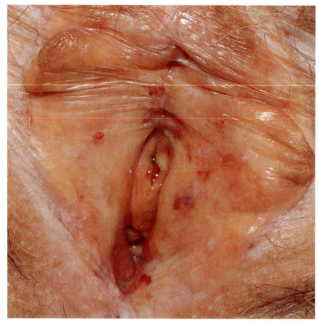

Fig. 3.70   Lichen sclerosus. An example of marked loss of tissue, telangiectasia and purpura.

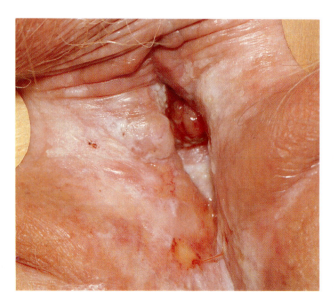

Fig. 3.71   Lichen sclerosus. A similar example, where the situation may have been aggravated by previous X-ray therapy.

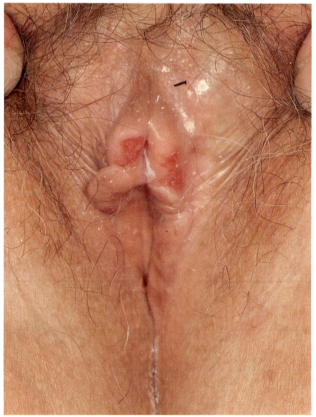

Fig. 3.72   Lichen sclerosus. A patient with persistent periclitoral erosion, in whom a carcinoma developed in the area on the left.

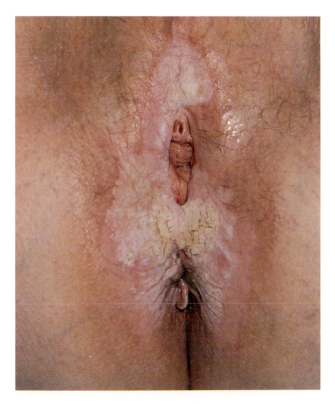

Fig. 3.73 Lichen sclerosus. Hyperkeratotic plaque in a patient who has had a vulvectomy for malignancy. Repeated biopsies showed no evidence of malignancy. The lesion recurred after laser and after excision but is now kept in a soft and symptomless state by the occasional use of a potent typical corticosteroid.

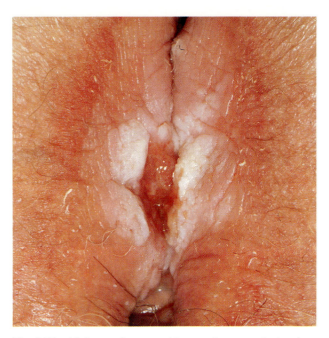

Fig. 3.74 Lichen sclerosus. After a vulvectomy for benign disease, this patient developed a carcinoma in the middle of an apparently similar hyperkeratotic plaque.

VULVODYNIA

The term 'vulvodynia' is used for a complaint of chronic burning and soreness. A statement of current views of its nature and subdivisions is given in Appendix B. Patients with essential dysaesthetic vulvodynia have no abnormal physical signs. There are two groups of patients with unequivocal signs, those with vestibular papillomatosis and those with the vulval vestibulitis syndrome.

Vestibular papillomatosis

A few papillary lesions are visible in the posterior part of the vestibule in many women; these appear to be a variant of normal. In papillomatosis, which may or may not be symptomatic, the inner aspects of the labia minora and the vestibule are covered with tiny papillae, clearly visible to the naked eye (Fig. 3.76). The surface shows aceto-whitening but the change is not now thought to be consistently associated with HPV infection—the effect of acetic acid is probably non-specific. Those who have no symptoms should by definition be excluded from the category of vulvodynia.

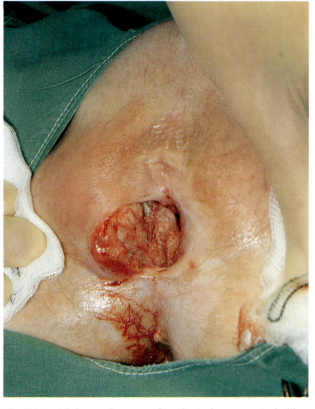

Fig. 3.75 Lichen sclerosus. A patient who presented with a carcinoma was found to have symptomless lichen sclerosus.

Vulval vestibulitis

Patients complain of pain on touch and pressure in localized areas within the vestibule. Their usual complaints are therefore related to tampon insertion and to sexual intercourse. Patchy erythema is usually found at these areas which are exquisitely tender on pressure. The erythema may be almost punctate or quite diffuse and lesions may be single or (more usually) multiple (Figs 3.77–3.80). Occasionally there is deposition of haemosiderin, giving the red areas a brownish hue. In such cases the lesions clinically resemble what has been termed Zoon's vulvitis (the female equivalent of Zoon's balanitis), although some feel that this diagnosis should be reserved for cases showing certain histological features. The exact status of Zoon's vulvitis in relation to vestibulitis, where the histology is non-specific, is at present uncertain.

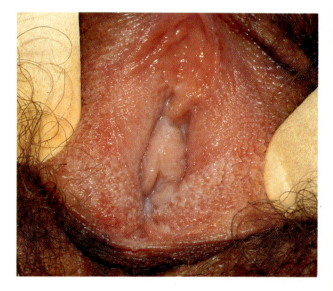

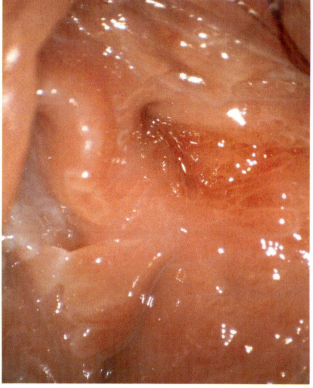

Fig. 3.76 Vestibular papillomatosis. The vestible and inner aspects of the labia minora are covered with papillae. The appearance will be accentuated by the application of acetic acid.

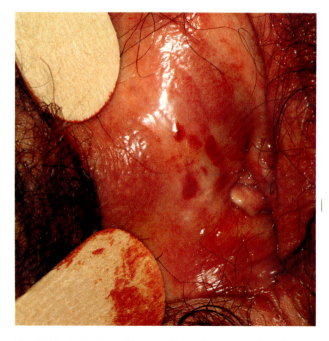

Fig. 3.77 Vulval vestibulitis. Extensive areas of erythema that are tender on point pressure.

Fig. 3.78 Vulval vestibulitis. An area of erythema near the opening of Bartholin's gland duct.

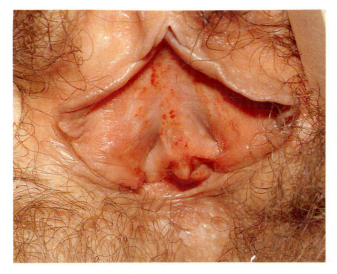

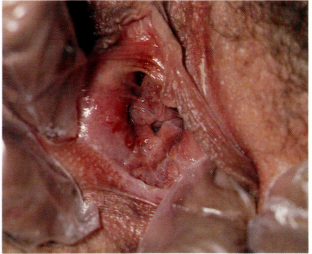

Fig. 3.79   Vulval vestibulitis. Tender punctate areas. Histology non-specific.

Fig. 3.80   Vulval vestibulitis. Tender punctate areas and some haemosiderin pigment. Histology non-specific.

4. *Tumour-like Lesions and Cysts, and Tumours*

TUMOUR-LIKE LESIONS AND CYSTS

It cannot be emphasized too strongly that unless the clinical diagnosis of a benign lesion, which can be safely left alone, is absolutely certain, all lesions of this type should be either biopsied or excised for histological examination.

Ectopic tissue, for example breast tissue or endometriosis (Fig. 4.1), may mimic a neoplasm.

Cysts may be developmental or epidermoid or may

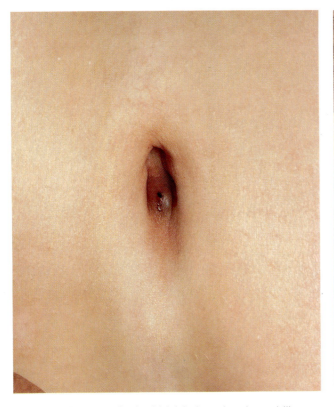

Fig. 4.1 Endometriosis. A bluish deposit at the umbilicus.

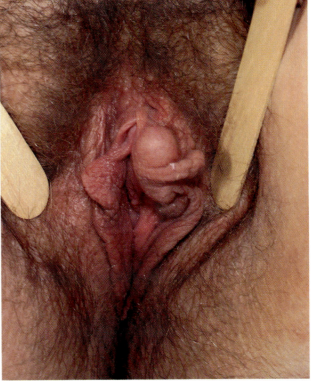

Fig. 4.2 This cyst, arising laterally in the vulva, is of mesonephric origin.

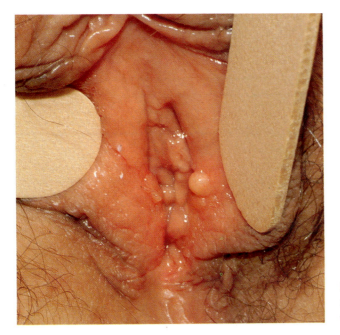

Fig. 4.3 Mucinous cyst. Arising in the vestibule from a minor vestibular gland or from dysontogenic urogenital sinus epithelium.

develop as a result of a blockage of the gland ducts (Figs 4.2–4.5). The position and the histology of the cyst will enable it to be categorized. Bartholin's cysts are initially acute and painful and their site is diagnostic.

NON-EPITHELIAL TUMOURS

A variety of these mesenchymal tumours may present at the vulva as tumours which are benign or malignant (sarcomas). The fibroma usually found on the labia majora (Fig. 4.6) is an example of a benign lesion.

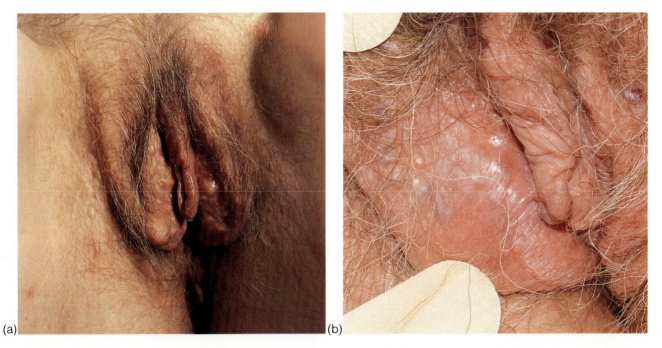

(a)　　　　　　　　　　　　　　　　　　　(b)

Fig. 4.4　Cyst. This type of cyst may be primary epidermoid or may develop from squamous metaplasia in the ducts of the sebaceous glands. The patient's usual complaint is of the appearance. A similar clinical picture may develop through blockage of the ducts.

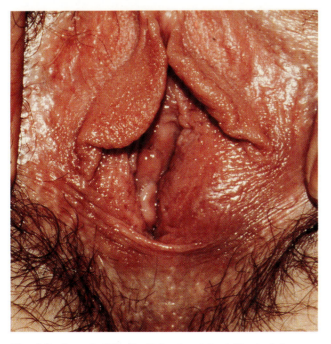

Fig. 4.5　A cyst of Bartholin's gland duct. The bulging area is seen on one side.

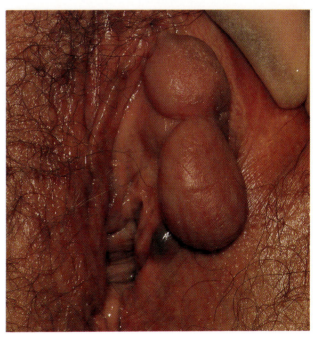

Fig. 4.6　Labial fibromas.

Haemangiomas

Haemangiomas of cavernous type are confined to childhood.

Angiokeratomas

Small angiokeratomas are common in adults and are found mainly on the labia majora. They present as small red or dark punctate or rather larger lesions and are single or multiple (Fig. 4.7). The darkness of solitary lesions may result in their being mistaken for a melanoma (Fig. 4.8) or other lesion (Fig. 4.9). Small multiple lesions can be difficult to distinguish from the speckling often seen in lichen sclerosus.

Treatment is by excision, cautery or laser.

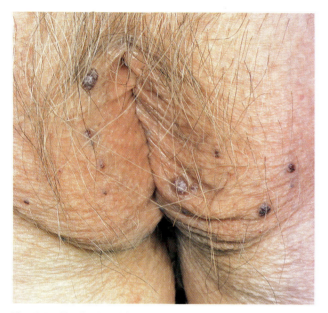

Fig. 4.7 Typical multiple angiokeratomas.

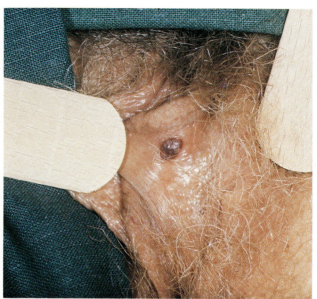

Fig. 4.8 A solitary angiokeratoma.

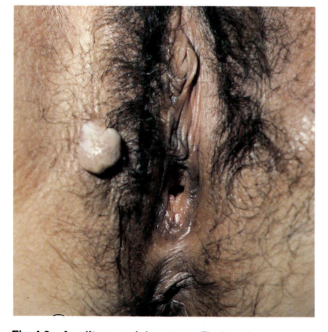

Fig. 4.9 A solitary angiokeratoma. The keratinous covering made the clinical diagnosis difficult.

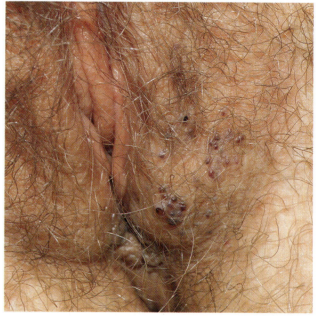

Fig. 4.10 Lymphangioma. The frogspawn-like appearance of these lesions, their early onset and the unilateral distribution, makes the diagnosis of lymphangioma probable.

Lymphangiomas

Lymphangiomas may not be truly neoplastic. Lymphangioma circumscriptum has small frogspawn-like vesicles (Fig. 4.10) and, because of connection with deep lymphatic cisterns, local destruction may result in recurrence. Lymphoedema and lymphangiectasia are noted elsewhere (see p. 78).

Granular cell tumour

Granular cell tumours arise from Schwann cells and the vulva is a site of election, although the lesion is uncommon. Neurofibroma and fibroma must be considered in the differential diagnosis (Fig. 4.11).

Sarcoma and lymphoma

Sarcoma and lymphoma may occur but they are rare.

EPITHELIAL TUMOURS

Benign epithelial tumours

The common benign epithelial tumours are viral warts, non-viral squamous papillomas, skin tags (Figs 4.12 and 4.13) and basal cell papillomas (Fig. 4.14). If the diagnosis is definite the non-infective ones can be left alone, but removal is usually simple and satisfactory.

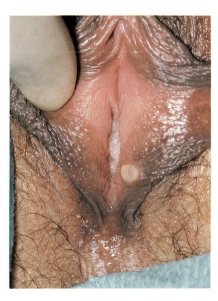

Fig. 4.11 A granular cell tumour of the vulva. A firm yellowish nodule.

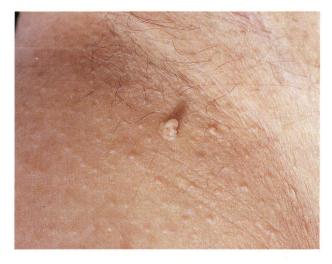

Fig. 4.12 A skin tag (fibro-epithelial polyp) in the groin.

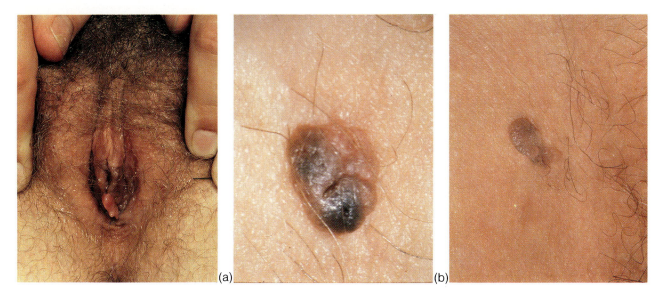

(a)   (b)

Fig. 4.13 This tag-like lesion is a hymenal remnant.

Fig. 4.14 (a), (b) Basal cell papilloma (seborrhoeic wart). A dark, warty superficial plaque.

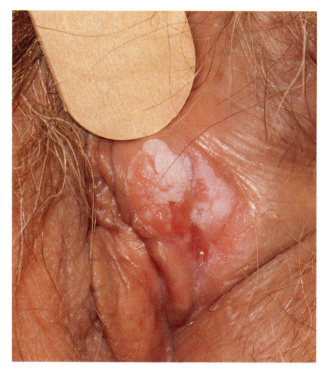

Fig. 4.15 Vulval intra-epithelial neoplasia. The main complaint of the patient in Fig. 4.14 (b) was this fixed eroded patch, seen medially. Histology showed vulvar intra-epithelial neoplasm.

Vulval intra-epithelial neoplasia

Vulval intra-epithelial neoplasia (VIN) does not present as a tumour and may superficially resemble benign dermatoses (Fig. 4.15). It is classified as squamous and non-squamous.

Squamous VIN

The squamous form of VIN has a strikingly pleomorphic appearance—it may be red, white, pigmented, warty, moist or eroded. The whole of the vulva, perineum and peri-anal area may be involved (Figs 4.16–4.20). VIN 1 and 2 (see Appendix A) are difficult to differentiate from HPV lesions. Full-thickness changes—VIN 3 or carcinoma *in situ*—are of clinical consequence and are illustrated here. When this condition is diagnosed it is important to examine the whole of the lower genital tract and anal canal, and to keep them under subsequent observation, because lesions in other parts, particularly the cervix, are common and usually of greater importance than the vulval lesions.

Treatment of VIN is controversial. In a non-immuno-suppressed patient there is a case for minimal intervention if supervision is close. Lesions in pregnancy will often regress after the birth. However,

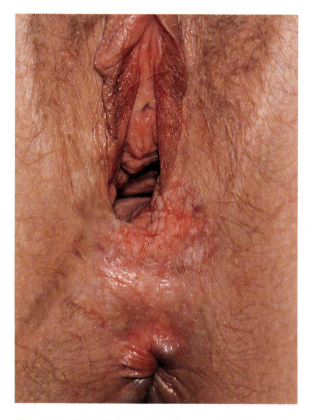

Fig. 4.16 Vulval intra-epithelial neoplasia. Presenting as a reddish lesion in the perineum.

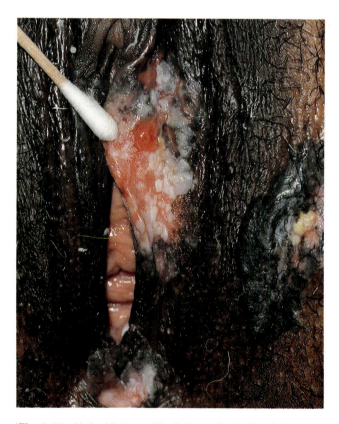

Fig. 4.17 Vulval intra-epithelial neoplasia. Eroded white and red plaque in a dark-skinned patient.

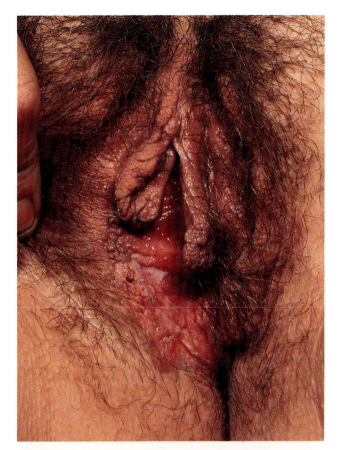

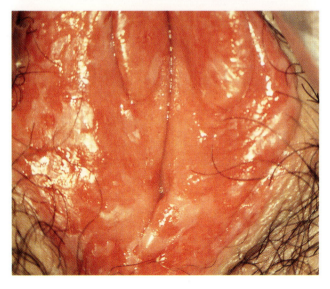

Fig. 4.18 Vulval intra-epithelial neoplasia. Examples showing eroded erythema. Histological examination is required to distinguish this from erosive lichen planus or other erosive dermatoses.

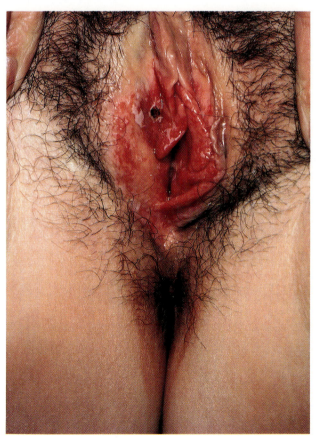

judicious use of wide local excision and the laser are usually successful when lesions are extensive and give rise to symptoms. It is important whatever course is chosen to be prepared to check on multiple histological specimens so that foci of invasion are likely to be disclosed.

Non-squamous VIN

Non-squamous VIN—extramammary Paget's disease—may be localized or widespread. The lesions are red, moist or scaly. The resemblance to a banal dermatosis is often close (Figs 4.21 and 4.22).

Treatment is essentially surgical. The points to bear in mind are that pathological changes tend to extend beyond the clinical borders and that in some cases (about 25 per cent) there is an underlying neoplasm, and/or neoplasia elsewhere in the anogenital area or breasts.

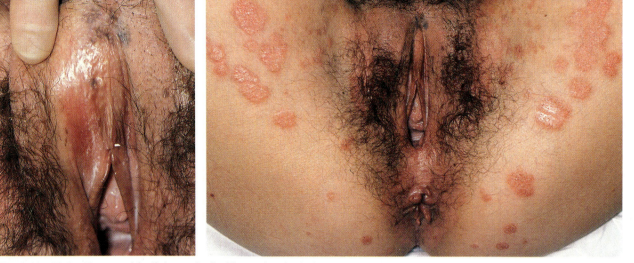

Fig. 4.19   Vulval intra-epithelial neoplasia. The patient had pigmented macular lesions anteriorly (the patient also had psoriasis).

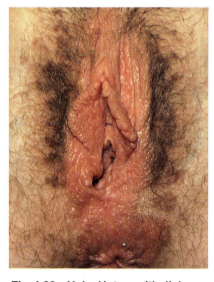

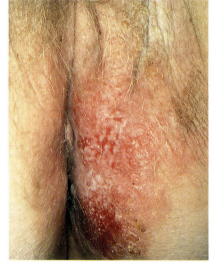

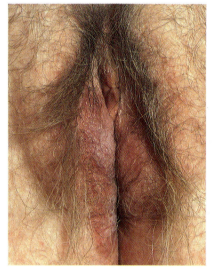

Fig. 4.20   Vulval intra-epithelial neoplasia. Pigmented warty lesions. This is a clinical picture and may be termed 'Bowenoid papulosis'. This term should not be used to imply a histological diagnosis.

Fig. 4.21   Extramammary Paget's disease. Extensive lesions that had recurred following excision over several years.

Fig. 4.22   Extramammary Paget's disease. Lesion on patient's right. This patient presented with a non-specific, itching, thickened patch. Its lack of response over 2–3 weeks to a topical corticosteroid showed the need for a biopsy and this established the diagnosis of extramammary Paget's disease.

Malignant epithelial tumours

Squamous cell carcinoma

Much the most common malignant tumour is squamous cell carcinoma. The pruritic, ulcerated or hard lesions, often bleeding, are usually easy to recognize. They may arise on a background of VIN (Fig. 4.23), lichen sclerosus (Fig. 4.24) or from apparently normal tissue (Fig. 4.25).

Variants of squamous cell carcinoma, such as adeno-squamous carcinoma and adenocarcinoma, can occur but the diagnosis is made on histological, not clinical, grounds.

Treatment is essentially surgical and vulvectomy, usually with bilateral inguinal lymphadenectomy, is the accepted mode. Pelvic lymphadenectomy is usually carried out only when the tumour is large or when there are clearly extensively involved nodes.

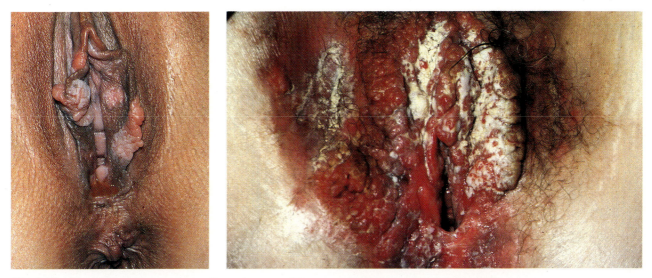

Fig. 4.23 Examples of squamous cell carcinoma arising on vulval intra-epithelial neoplasia.

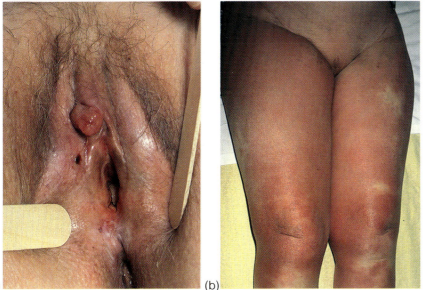

(a)   (b)

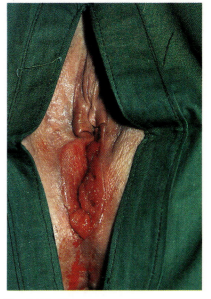

Fig. 4.24 **(a) Squamous cell carcinoma arising on lichen sclerosus.** This was noted only when the patient presented with the lump; it had previously been symptomless. **(b) Severe cellulitis** following vulvectomy in the patient shown in (a). Cellulitis is a well-recognised hazard of radical vulvectomy because of residual lymphoedema.

Fig. 4.25 **Squamous cell carcinoma.** Without evidence of underlying vulval intra-epithelial neoplasia or lichen sclerosus.

Verrucous carcinoma

Verrucous carcinoma is uncommon, clinically malignant but histologically benign. It may be related to infection with HPV 6 and 11 (Fig. 4.26). The lesion resembles (or may be) a giant condylomata acuminatum—relentlessly growing and extending.

Treatment is by vulvectomy.

Basal cell carcinomas

Basal cell carcinomas may occur at the vulva and take the form of solid nodules, not resembling the superficial type seen on other covered areas (Fig. 4.27).

Treatment is by simple local excision.

Melanocytic lesions

Benign melanocytic lesions

Moles are not uncommon at the vulva and may be junctional, compound or intradermal (Fig. 4.28). Rarer types peculiar to the vulva may be seen. Excision is recommended, as elsewhere, if there are any features of malignancy.

Lentigines are macular melanocytic lesions and may be solitary or multiple (Fig. 4.29). They are characterized by an increased number of normal melanocytes along the dermo-epidermal junction with many melanophages in the papillary body. Larger areas of confluent pigmentation with similar benign histological features are now referred to as melanosis (Fig. 4.30). Without histological examination these changes can be difficult to differentiate from pigmented VIN and postinflammatory hyperpigmentation. In doubtful cases biopsy is essential.

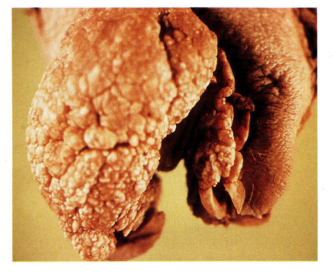

Fig. 4.26   A verrucous carcinoma.

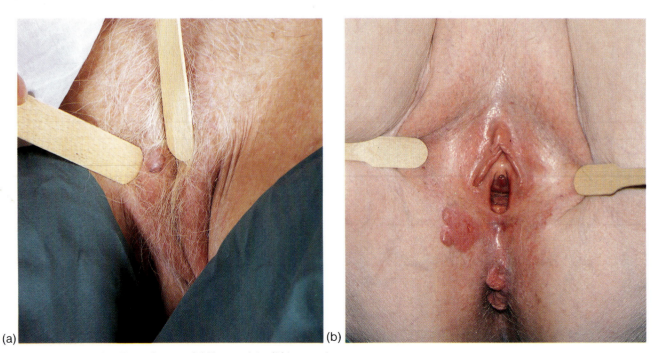

(a)

(b)

Fig. 4.27   Basal cell carcinoma. (a) Firm nodule. **(b)** Large plaque.

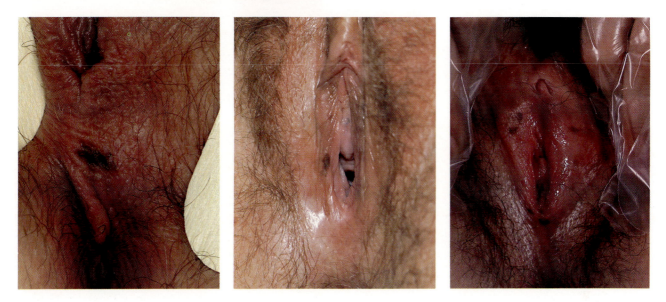

Fig. 4.28 **Mole.** A soft brown fleshy nodule.

Fig. 4.29 **Lentigo.** Examples of typical dark macules. Biopsy is essential to distinguish them from pigmented vulval intra-epithelial neoplasia.

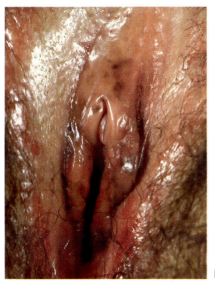

Fig. 4.30 **Melanosis.** More diffuse and extensive intensely dark pigmentation.

Malignant melanoma

Malignant melanoma may arise *de novo* or from a pre-existing lesion, and it may be of the superficial spreading or nodular variety (Figs 4.31–4.33). It may involve any area of the vulva and, although it may be amelanotic, is usually pigmented.

It is clearly important to recognize this lesion which, although rare, is highly malignant and often diagnosed at a late stage. Ulceration and bleeding are common presenting complaints.

Prognosis, as in malignant melanoma elsewhere, is closely related to the depth of the lesion. Treatment is surgical; recent trends favour wide local excision as with malignant melanoma elsewhere rather than routine vulvectomy.

Adnexal neoplasms

Benign syringomas (Fig. 4.34)—related to eccrine sweat glands and presenting as single or numerous skin-coloured papules—and benign hidradenomas—larger, usually solitary swellings related to apocrine sweat glands—are examples of adnexal neoplasms.

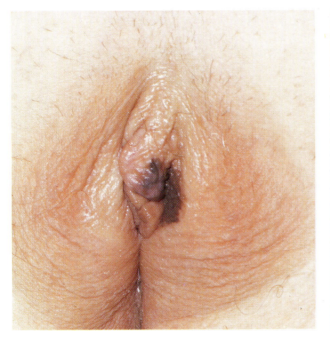

Fig. 4.31 Melanoma. An example of the superficial spreading variety.

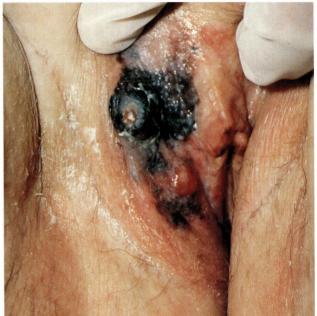

Fig. 4.32 Melanoma.

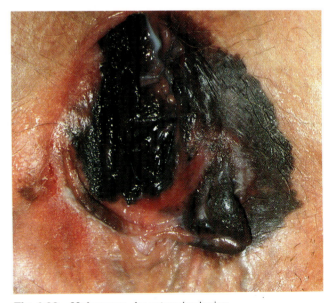

Fig. 4.33 Melanoma. An extensive lesion.

Other rare adnexal tumours are seen from time to time, as are their malignant counterparts.

The urethra and Bartholin's gland and duct may be the site of benign and malignant tumours (hence the importance of establishing histological evidence when operating on the rare Bartholin's abscesses in older women).

Metastatic tumours

Metastatic tumours may arise at the vulva, presenting as single or multiple dermal or subcutaneous masses (Fig. 4.35). Their most common origin is from primary neoplasms of the cervix, endometrium, vagina, ovary, urethra, kidney, breast, rectum or lung.

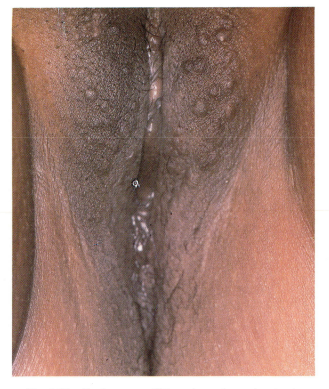

Fig. 4.34 Syringomas. Skin-coloured papules. Lesions are usually present elsewhere.

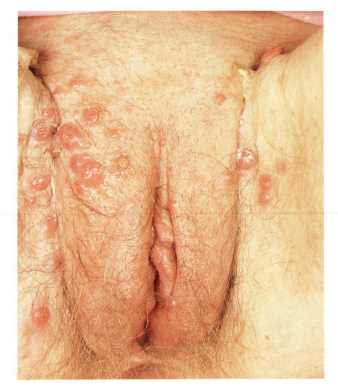

Fig. 4.35 Metastatic tumours. Secondary deposits from an ovarian carcinoma.

5. Miscellaneous Conditions

Chronic lymphoedema may be primary (Fig. 5.1) — related to congenital lymphatic hypoplasia — or secondary. Secondary forms arise from filariasis or from obstruction caused by surgery and radiotherapy, or in Crohn's disease (Fig. 5.2). Vesicles (lymphangiectasia) develop in long-standing cases (Fig. 5.3); these can be mistaken for condylomata acuminata. In other cases, repeated attacks of cellulitis occur. Laser treatment may help the lymphangiectasia and long-term penicillin or erythromycin controls the cellulitis.

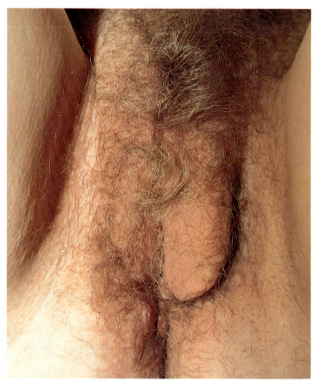

Fig. 5.1   Primary lymphoedema. No underlying reason for this chronic swelling could be found.

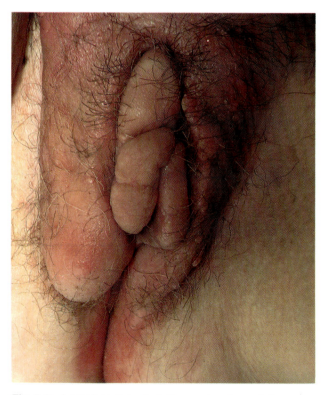

Fig. 5.2   Lymphoedema in inflammatory bowel disease. This patient was subject to repeated attacks of cellulitis.

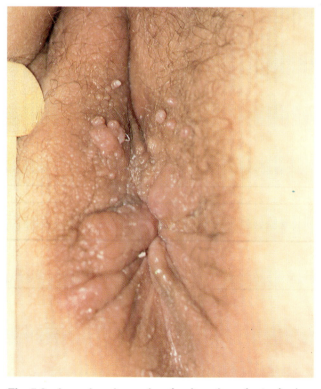

Fig. 5.3   Lymphoedema showing lymphangiectasia. A girl of 17 with oral lesions suggestive of Crohn's disease but who as yet shows no evidence of bowel involvement.

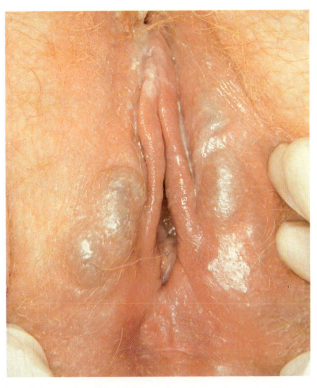

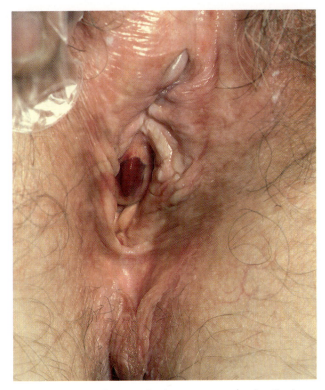

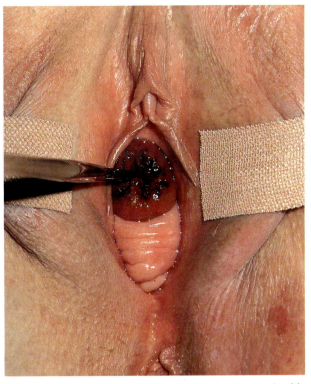

VARICOSITIES OF THE VULVA

Varicosities of the vulva are common in pregnancy and can arise in the first trimester; they also arise in chronic pelvic obstruction or portal hypertension in the middle-aged or elderly (Fig. 5.4).

URETHRAL CARUNCLE

In its milder forms this red swelling is very common and represents everted and inflamed urethral mucosa. More severe examples may be painful and bleeding and, in these cases, simple treatment with cautery is beneficial (Fig. 5.5).

URETHRAL PROLAPSE

Prolapsed tissue presents as an engorged reddened mass and must be distinguished from a tumour (Fig. 5.6).

Fig. 5.4   Varicosities of the vulva. The patient was 38 weeks pregnant. Such varices usually remit after delivery.

Fig. 5.5   Urethral caruncle. A postmenopausal patient (who also had lichen sclerosus). The lesion is red, painful and may bleed. It is part of the urethral mucosa but may be mistaken for a neoplasm.

Fig. 5.6   Urethral prolapse. As with a urethral caruncle, this may be mistaken for a neoplasm.

79

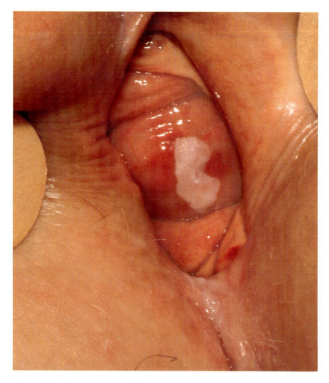

Fig. 5.7 **Cystocoele.** With hyperkeratotic area developing on mucosa.

CYSTOCOELE, PROLAPSE OF THE CERVIX, RECTOCOELE AND PROCIDENTIA

Cystocoele (Fig. 5.7), prolapse of the cervix (Fig. 5.8), rectocoele (Fig. 5.9) and procidentia are usually easily recognized.

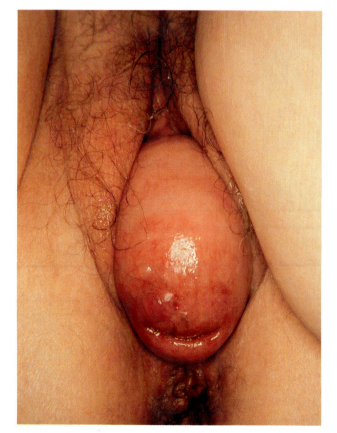

Fig. 5.8 **Prolapse of cervix.**

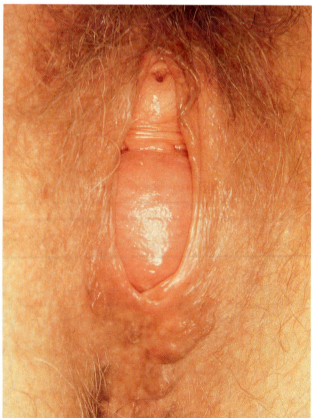

Fig. 5.9 **Rectocoele.**

RADIO-NECROSIS

Radio-necrosis is now seen only very occasionally. It was a complication of earlier methods of radiotherapy used for carcinoma of the vulva (Fig. 5.10).

RADIODERMATITIS

Radiodermatitis is occasionally encountered in patients with lichen sclerosus whose intractable pruritus was treated with radiation in pre-topical corticosteroid days (Fig. 5.11). Radiation damage predisposes to malignancy and such patients should be kept under review.

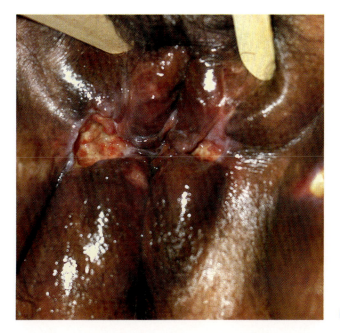

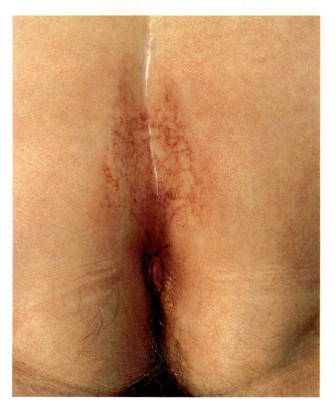

Fig. 5.10   Radiation necrosis. Ulcers.

Fig. 5.11   Radiodermatitis in a patient who had radiotherapy for pruritus of lichen sclerosus.

TRAUMATIC LESIONS

Traumatic lesions may be accidental, related to surgical procedures (Figs 5.12 and 5.13), or occasionally artefactual, a consequence of sexual abuse in a child (see Chapter 7) or rape in the adult. In the case of rape, expert examination for forensic evidence and to explore the possibility of sexually transmitted disease is essential.

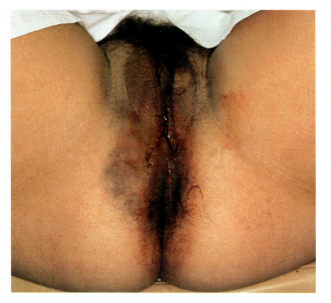

Fig. 5.12 Haematoma on right following episiotomy.

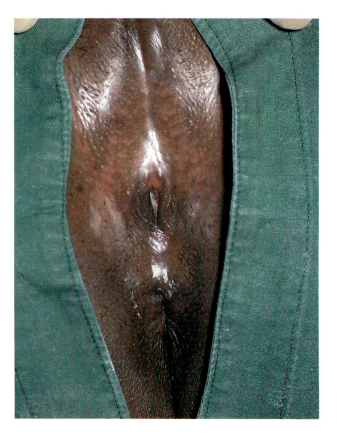

Fig. 5.13 Alteration of normal anatomy of vulva following a circumcision operation.

6. Childhood Lesions

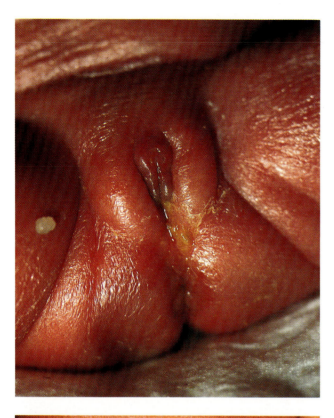

At birth, and for a few weeks afterwards, the vulval tissues are under the influence of maternal and placental hormones and appear puffy and engorged (Fig. 6.1).

The labia minora are prominent until puberty, when the labia majora develop. Labial adhesions may appear, usually in the first few months of life, and can be freed by surgical separation, oestrogen creams or bland emollients; spontaneous separation may be awaited (Fig. 6.2). Labial adhesions sometimes give rise to suspicion of ambiguous genitalia—a very rare finding. Figures 6.3–6.5 show ambiguous genitalia of different origins but with similar phenotypes, which cannot be distinguished on clinical examination. The importance of swift referral to an expert gynaecologist or paediatrician is self-evident.

Imperforate hymen will become apparent some 3 years after the menarche, presenting with primary amenorrhoea, abdominal pain and haematocolpos (Fig. 6.6).

Fig. 6.1   Engorgement of the vulva in a neonate. This patient also had staphylococcal scalded skin syndrome.

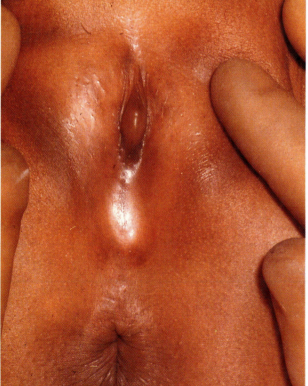

Fig. 6.2   Labial adhesions. A pinhole meatus is left anteriorly. The adhesions can be separated and kept apart by bland creams or oestrogen creams and spontaneous resolution is, in any case, common. The differential diagnosis is from fusion in lichen sclerosus.

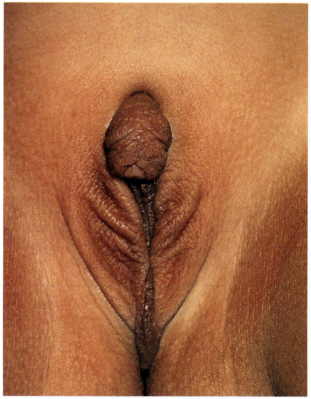

Fig. 6.3   Ambiguous genitalia in a boy. 5-alpha-reductase deficiency.

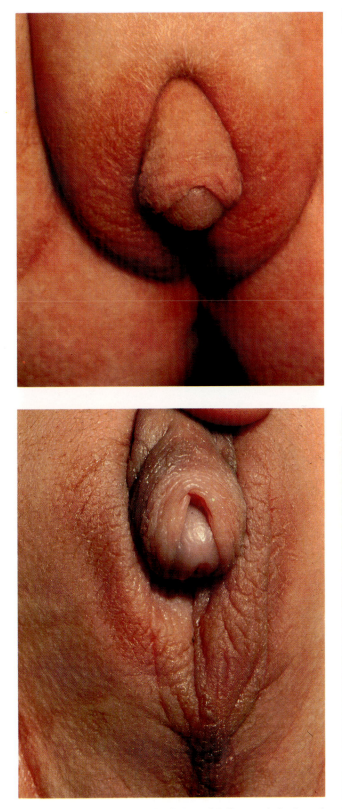

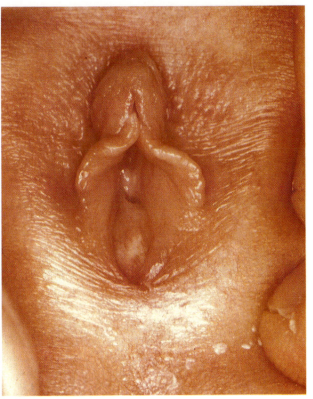

Fig. 6.4   Ambiguous genitalia in a girl. 21-hydroxylase deficiency.

Fig. 6.5   Ambiguous genitalia in a girl. Congenital adrenal hyperplasia as a result of 11-beta-hydroxylase deficiency.

Fig. 6.6   Imperforate hymen. This condition will come to light after the menarche when the tissue will bulge in front of accumulated menstrual blood.

NAPKIN RASH

Napkin rashes are common in infancy. The most common form, the primary irritant type, spares the folds and is diffuse. The changes are often most marked at the edges of the area. Secondary infection with bacteria and *Candida* is frequent. Pigmentary changes readily supervene in dark-skinned infants and these must be distinguished from the depigmentation of vitiligo (Fig. 6.7). In some cases shallow eroded areas develop with prominent edges (Fig. 6.8).

Seborrhoeic napkin rash tends to be red, dry and

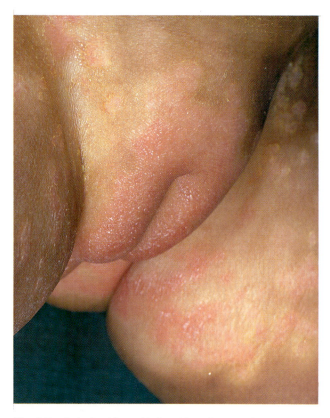

Fig. 6.7   A dark-skinned infant showing patchy hypopigmentation following a napkin rash. The parents can be reassured that the changes will right themselves.

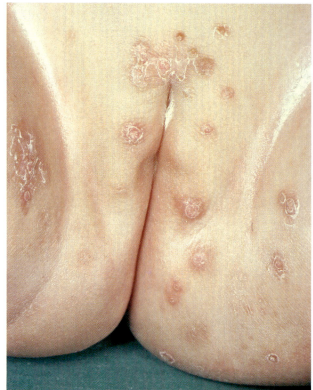

Fig. 6.8   Napkin rash. Shallow eroded areas.

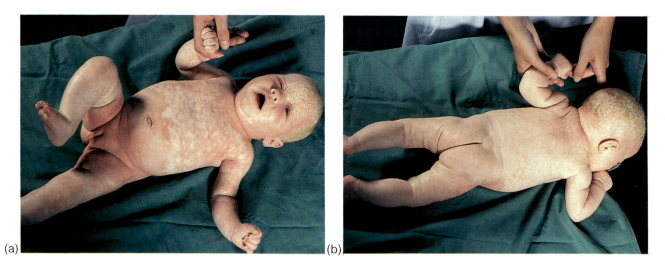

(a)

(b)

Fig. 6.9   Seborrhoeic napkin rash. (a) and (b) Redness of napkin area with extensive lesions elsewhere. Note the thick 'cradle cap' on the scalp.

scaly, and to be associated with lesions elsewhere, particularly of the scalp and face, and behind the ears (Fig. 6.9).

Psoriasiform napkin rashes feature scaly, well-defined patches in the napkin area and elsewhere (Fig. 6.10). In some cases true psoriasis is probably trig-

gered off by a primary irritant napkin rash but in the main the psoriasiform eruption does not imply a true psoriatic diathesis. Atopic dermatitis occasionally affects the napkin area.

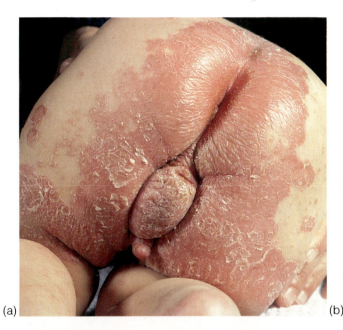
(a)

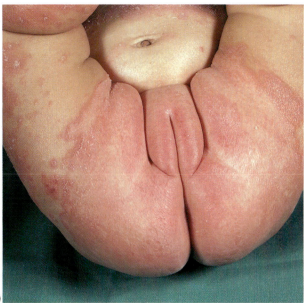
(b)

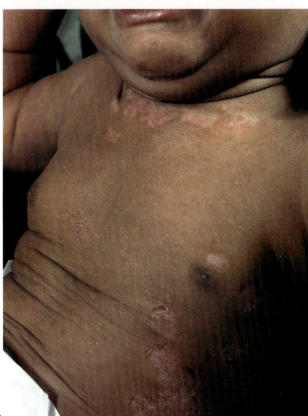
(c)

Fig. 6.10 Napkin psoriasis. (a) and (b) Well-defined red scaly areas in napkin areas in males and females. **(c)** Psoriasiform lesions on the trunk.

Two rare conditions – acrodermatitis enteropathica (Fig. 6.11) and Langerhans cell histiocytosis (Fig. 6.12) (histiocytosis X; Letterer-Siwe disease) – have a predilection for the vulval area in infancy and must be considered in the differential diagnosis.

Effective management of napkin rash depends upon keeping the area open and dry as far as possible.

Napkins should be well-rinsed. Bland emollients together with mild corticosteroids and antibacterial and anti-*Candida* agents are helpful.

BULLOUS DISEASE

Cases of Stevens–Johnson syndrome, pemphigoid and cicatricial pemphigoid have been reported in childhood but all are rare. The main (but still rare) cause of bullae at the anogenital area in childhood is chronic bullous disease of childhood — linear IgA disease and its more severe form childhood cicatricial pemphigoid. In cicatricial pemphigoid the ocular mucosa is often involved.

The bullae are subepidermal and show linear IgA at the basement membrane zone on direct im-

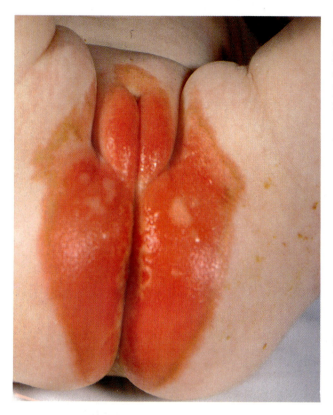

Fig. 6.11 Zinc deficiency. Typical fiery eroded erythema of the napkin area. The child was premature, a feature predisposing to this condition. The appearance is identical to that of the genetically determined acrodermatitis enteropathica.

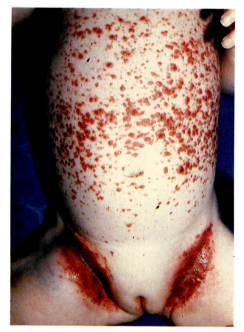

Fig. 6.12 Langerhans cell histiocytosis (histiocytosis X: Letterer-Siwe disease. Dusky purpuric papules in the napkin area, in this case accompanied by lesions elsewhere.

munofluorescence. Bullae occur on the trunk and limbs but have a predilection for the anogenital area (Fig. 6.13). The condition responds to oral dapsone or sulfapyridine; the latter is better tolerated in childhood.

PSORIASIS AND ECZEMA

Psoriasis and eczema are unusual at the vulva in childhood. Their features remain typical (Fig. 6.14).

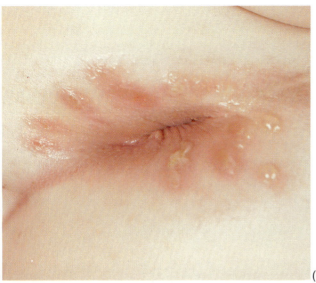

(a)

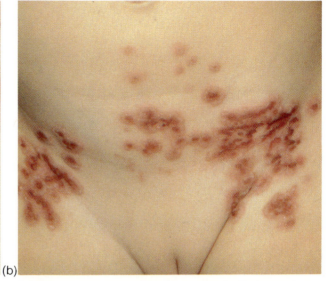

(b)

Fig. 6.13   Chronic bullous disease of childhood (linear IgA disease). (a) Tense bullae in the peri-anal area.

(b) Bullae on the trunk. The lesions are typically grouped together forming 'clusters of jewels'.

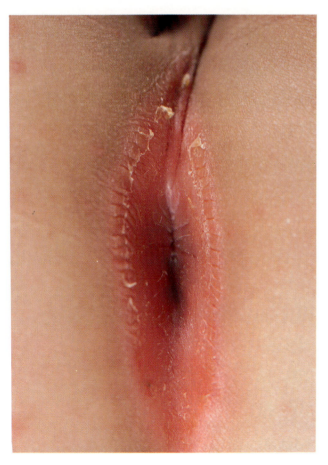

Fig. 6.14   A patch of psoriasis at the anal area. This child had typical psoriasis of the scalp and nails.

LICHEN SCLEROSUS

Lichen sclerosus (lichen sclerosus et atrophicus) is far from uncommon in childhood. It presents a wide variety of appearances ranging from tiny localized white or telangiectatic areas to florid changes with purpura—blood blisters—and frank bleeding in association with atrophy and loss of substance. The vulva and peri-anal area are usually involved together (Figs 6.15 and 6.16). Lichen sclerosus may be symptomless but often causes itching and soreness. Dysuria and constipation are common problems and if the underlying skin disease is not recognized they may lead to unnecessary investigation and treatment.

The main differential diagnoses are banal infective lesions, child sexual abuse and vitiligo (Fig. 6.17). Bland emollients and topical corticosteroids, with treatment of secondary infection as necessary, are effective. Mild corticosteroids are quite safe but the justification for using very potent corticosteroids in the hope of preventing loss of tissue is still under review. The condition tends to improve with time but probably does not resolve completely; symptoms remit and patients tend to be lost to follow-up, hence uncertainty in advising on prognosis.

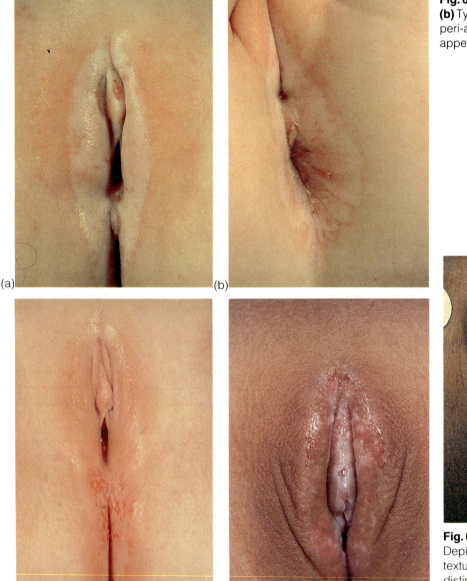

(a)   (b)

Fig. 6.15   Lichen sclerosus. (a) and (b) Typical appearance at vulva and in peri-anal area. Note the pallor and shiny appearance.

Fig. 6.16   Lichen sclerosus with marked infection and inflammation.

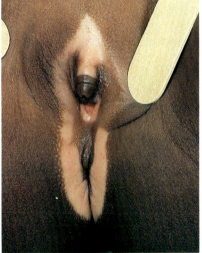

Fig. 6.17   Vitiligo in a child. Depigmentation with no change of texture—features that serve to distinguish it from postinflammatory hypopigmentation and from the pallor of lichen sclerosus, which is accompanied by atrophy.

INFECTIONS

Warts, herpes and molluscum contagiosum affect the vulva and peri-anal area (Figs 6.18 and 6.19). Acquisition may be by sexual or non-sexual means. Treatment of the lesions is as in adults, although general anaesthesia may be required to deal with warts.

Secondary infection of napkin rashes with bacteria and *Candida* is common.

Poor hygiene in later childhood may be associated with infection by staphylococci and streptococci, although streptococcal vulvitis sometimes occurs in healthy and clean children, possibly from a focus in the throat (Fig. 6.20). More often, staphylococci and, in particular, streptococci, infect already damaged skin, notably in lichen sclerosus. The infection may be recurrent. Management is with oral antibiotics and topical antiseptics, for example, povidone-iodine washes.

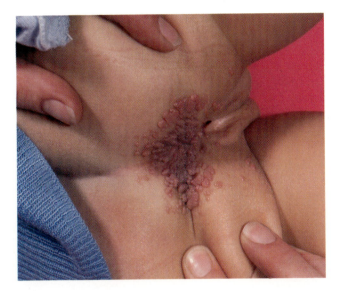

Fig. 6.18   Peri-anal warts.

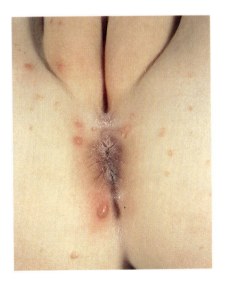

Fig. 6.19   Peri-anal molluscum contagiosum.

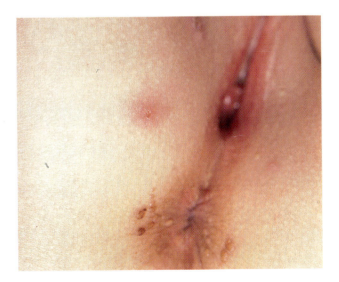

Fig. 6.20   A child with streptococcal vulvitis, warts and molluscum contagiosum.

Threadworm infestation leads to itching, redness and sometimes secondary infection; this is usually peri-anal but may be vulval. The diagnosis is made by taking early morning peri-anal sellotape swabs and treatment with piperazine of the whole family is essential to prevent reinfection. In any acute vulvitis or vulvovaginitis the possibility of a sexually transmitted disease, and hence of probable child sexual abuse, should be borne in mind.

NEOPLASIA

Malignant tumours

Malignant tumours, usually sarcomas, are rare and more often vaginal, presenting at the vulva, than of vulval origin.

Benign tumours

The most common benign tumours are moles and cavernous haemangiomas (Fig. 6.21).

If moles cause concern or show disquieting changes (rare before puberty) they should be observed and excised if necessary (Fig. 6.22).

Haemangiomas will resolve and should be left untreated unless they are of the rare giant type. Ulceration of these lesions is unusual and can be treated with simple applications and antibiotics as necessary.

TRAUMA

Straddle injuries and stretching that leads to tearing and accidental penetration are the main causes of accidental injury. Trauma in the form of scratching or minimal accidental injury will lead to purpura and frank bleeding in lichen sclerosus (Fig. 6.23). Child sexual abuse will often lead to injury.

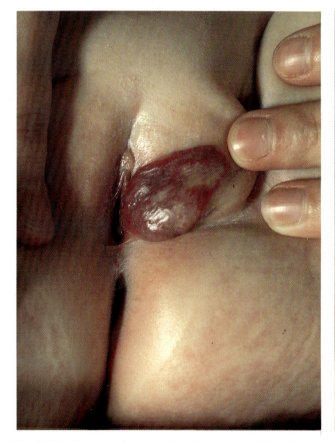
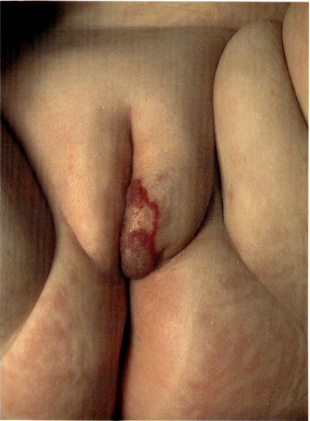

Fig. 6.21   Haemangioma of strawberry type at the vulva. This lesion occasionally bleeds and can become infected, but the prognosis is good.

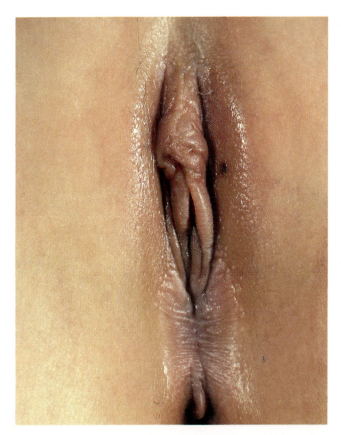

Fig. 6.22   Benign mole in a child (who also has lichen sclerosus).

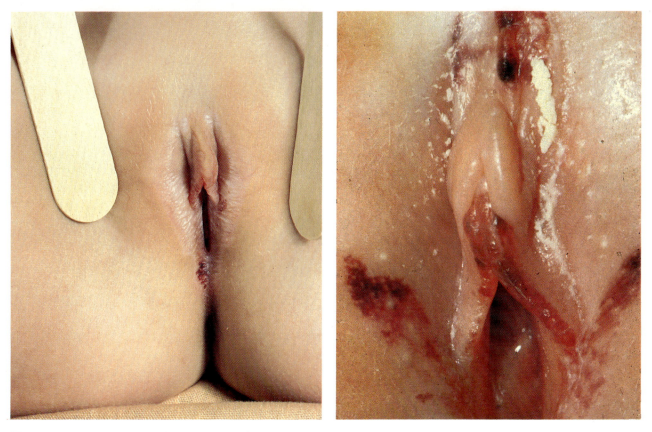

Fig. 6.23   Lichen sclerosus. Note the areas of purpura, which may lead to a mistaken diagnosis of sexual abuse.

7. Child Sexual Abuse

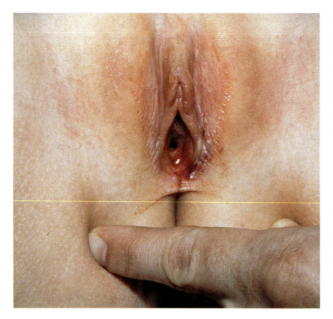

Fig. 7.1 Sexually abused 8-year-old girl. A tear of the posterior fourchette with bruising of the labia is visible. The dimension of the hymenal opening is within normal limits. Minimal discharge is present due to beta-haemolytic streptococcus.

Child sexual abuse (CSA) should be considered in the presence of suspicious physical signs, although there are often no abnormal physical findings, even when abuse has been established. The significance of physical signs should be assessed in the light of evidence that has been obtained by other means. They may support a child's statement of abuse or indicate a need for further investigation.

VULVAL EVIDENCE

Few signs are diagnostic of sexual abuse. However, in the absence of a reasonable alternative explanation, a laceration or scar on the hymen (Fig. 7.1), or of the anal mucosa extending beyond the anal verge onto the peri-anal skin, indicates that abuse has taken place.

The hymenal orifice dimension is not a reliable indicator of sexual abuse, although a horizontal diameter exceeding 1 cm in a prepubertal girl occurs more commonly after abuse and should arouse suspicion (Figs 7.2 and 7.3). The position of tears varies according to the type of abuse. Digital

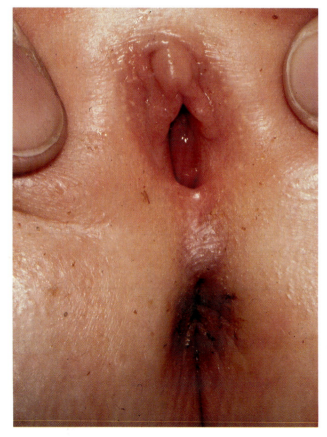

Fig. 7.2 A sexually abused child, aged 8. The hymenal orifice is widely dilated, with a thin rim of hymen persisting. There was a history of digital penetration.

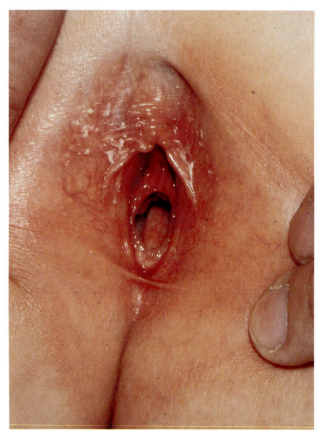

Fig. 7.3 Normal 18-month-old child. There is some normal reddening of the vulva. The fleshy hymen is typical of this age group. The anus is normal.

penetration tends to cause lacerations anteriorly whereas penile penetration is associated with tears of the posterior fourchette. Rubbing may produce symmetrical erythema of the vulval area (Fig. 7.4). The presence of bruising or scratches in adjacent areas would support the possibility of CSA.

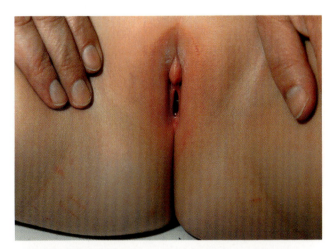

Fig. 7.4 Symmetrical vulval rash due to intracrural rubbing. Note the scratch marks visible on the buttocks. Sexual abuse was demonstrated.

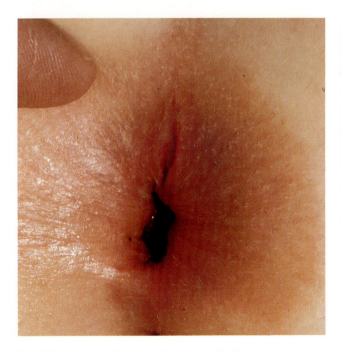

Fig. 7.5 A sexually abused girl, aged 6. The anus is lax and gaping, with a recent deep anal fissure posteriorly. The fissure extended 2 cm into the anal canal. There is some peri-anal reddening. There was a history of recent anal penetration—sodomy by the stepfather.

ANAL EVIDENCE

There are uncertainties within the profession over the significance of physical signs that may be due to conditions other than CSA; this is particularly so in the anal region (Fig. 7.5).

Erythema

Peri-anal erythema may occur in association with poor hygiene, irritation from threadworms and skin disorders but is commonly found in cases of abuse. The extent of erythema depends on the degree of friction.

Fissures

Anal fissures are not uncommon in children in whom there is no suspicion of abuse but these tend to be in the midline; multiple anal fissures should arouse suspicion of abuse.

Engorged veins

Engorged veins are common in small babies with constipation but venous congestion of the peri-anal plexus is often one of the last signs to resolve following anal abuse (Figs 7.6 and 7.7).

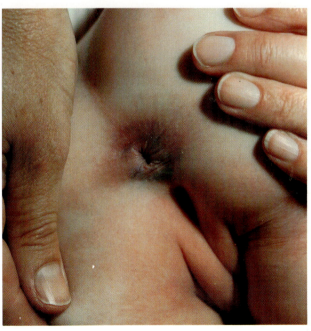

Fig. 7.6 Peri-anal venous engorgement and surrounding bruising of the anus in a sexually abused 3-year-old girl.

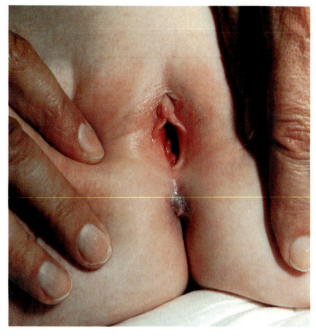

Fig. 7.7　A skin tag is visible and there is marked bruising. The diameter of the hymenal orifice is possibly increased with some surrounding oedema.

BACTERIAL INFECTION

Bacterial infection, particularly with organisms that may be sexually transmitted, raises the possibility of CSA.

Vulvitis caused by a bacterial infection has similar features, whether sexually or non-sexually transmitted, and it is important to establish a microbiological diagnosis in all cases (Fig. 7.8). Vulvovaginal swabs should be taken and placed in appropriate transport medium for culture of bacteria in the laboratory. This should include culture for *N. gonorrhoeae*, *Chlamydia trachomatis*, streptococci and staphylococci. Rectal swabs should be taken if anal abuse is suspected and, where there is clinical suspicion of other sexually transmitted diseases, e.g. herpes, syphilis, appropriate microbiological investigations should be performed (see Chapter 2).

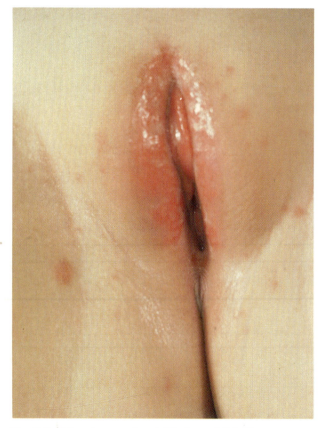

Fig. 7.8　Streptococcal vulvitis in a child. There was no evidence of sexual abuse.

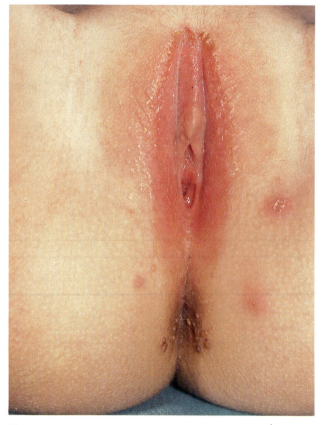

Fig. 7.9　A child with symmetrical vulval erythema and molluscum contagiosum. Note the presence of anal warts. These changes were not thought to be related to sexual abuse.

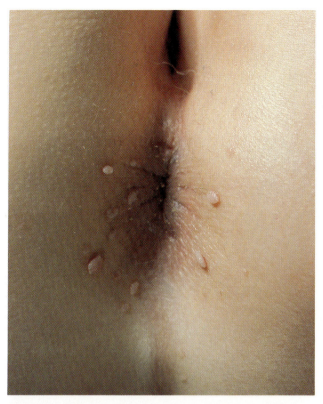

Fig. 7.10 Sessile warts visible in the peri-anal region.

WARTS

The presence of genital warts should also alert the physician to the possibility of abuse, although these may be acquired in other ways (Figs 7.9–7.11) (see p. 29).

Careful examination and investigation in suspected cases of CSA is mandatory as some conditions of the vulva may be mistaken for CSA. Inflammation, infection and purpura in lichen sclerosus in childhood may arouse suspicions about sexual abuse and the presence of the condition must not exclude abuse, as they may co-exist (Fig. 7.12).

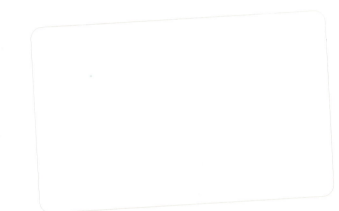

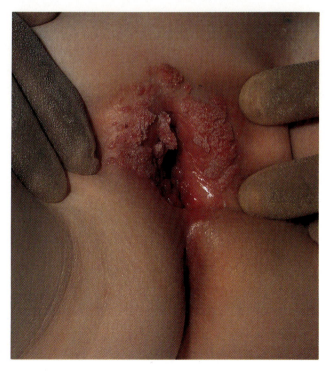

Fig. 7.11 Extensive perivulval wart infection in a 2-year-old child. Probable vertical transmission from the mother.

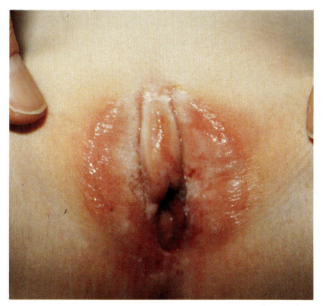

Fig. 7.12 9-year-old girl complaining of recurrent soreness. Child sexual abuse was established after a disclosure interview. There are signs of lichen sclerosus and associated infection with *Gardnerella vaginalis*, but these are not specific signs relating to sexual abuse.

Appendix A
Classification of Neoplastic and Non-neoplastic Conditions.

*International Society
for the Study
of Vulvar Disease
(ISSVD)*

VULVAL INTRA-EPITHELIAL NEOPLASIA (VIN) (ISSVD 1986)

Squamous VIN

1. VIN 1—mild dysplasia.
2. VIN 2—moderate dysplasia.
3. VIN 3—severe dysplasia or carcinoma *in situ*.

Non-squamous VIN

Paget's disease

NON-NEOPLASTIC EPITHELIAL DISORDERS OF VULVAL SKIN AND MUCOSA (ISSVD 1989)

1. Lichen sclerosus (Lichen sclerosus et atrophicus).
2. Squamous cell hyperplasia (formerly hyperplastic dystrophy).
3. Other dermatoses.

Mixed epithelial disorders may occur. In such cases it is recommended that both conditions be reported. For example, lichen sclerosus with associated squamous cell hyperplasia (formerly classified as mixed dystrophy) should be reported as lichen sclerosus and squamous cell hyperplasia. Squamous cell hyperplasia with associated vulval intra-epithelial neoplasia (formerly hyperplastic dystrophy with atypia) should be diagnosed as vulval intra-epithelial neoplasia.

Squamous cell hyperplasia is used for those instances in which the hyperplasia is not attributable to another cause. Specific lesions or dermatoses involving the vulva, e.g. psoriasis, lichen planus, lichen simplex chronicus, *Candida* infection and condyloma acuminatum, may include squamous cell hyperplasia but should be diagnosed specifically and excluded from this category.

Note This classification replaces that devised by the ISSVD in 1976, and which is given below for reference.

  I. Hyperplastic dystrophy:
    A. without atypia
    B. with atypia.
 II. Lichen sclerosus.
III. Mixed dystrophy (lichen sclerosus with foci of epithelial hyperplasia):
    A. without atypia
    B. with atypia.

REFERENCES

Ridley, C.M., Frankman, O., Jones, I.S.C. *et al.* (1989) New nomenclature for vulvar disease: ISSVD. *Human Pathol.*, **20**, 495–6.

Wilkinson, E.J., Kneale, B., Lynch, P.J. (1986) Report of the terminology committee. *J. Reprod. Med.*, **31**, 973–4.

Appendix B
Classification of vulvodynia (ISSVD)

VULVODYNIA*

Vulvodynia is chronic vulval discomfort, the patient complaining of burning or soreness but not itching. The term replaces 'burning vulva syndrome'.

Subgroups are now recognized and can be defined by certain criteria.

Vulval vestibulitis

Vulval vestibulitis is a chronic clinical syndrome that may be characterized by the following criteria:

1. Severe pain on vestibular touch or attempted vaginal entry.
2. Tenderness to pressure localized within the vulval vestibule.
3. Physical findings confined to vestibular erythema of various degrees.

As defined above, vulval vestibulitis does not include symptoms associated with acute inflammatory conditions or with immediate postoperative changes; these vulval symptoms resolve with appropriate therapy or after a reasonable period. The cause of vulval vestibulitis is not known, but the condition is thought to have a multifactorial aetiology. Local inflammation, irritation, and/or infection with bacteria, Candida or HPV have each been implicated in certain cases. It is also possible that the specialized epithelia of the vulval vestibule and minor vestibular glands may make this area particularly susceptible to morphological changes that may influence the development of vulvodynia.

Vestibular papillae have been described as tiny fibrillary growths in the vestibule, usually localized in the posterior portion; they are considered a normal anatomical variant.

Vestibular papillomatosis

Vestibular papillomatosis is a descriptive term for the presence of multiple papillae, which may cover the entire mucosal surface of the labia minora. Vestibular papillomatosis is sometimes seen with HPV infection but it should be emphasized that a consistent association has not been proved. Furthermore, papillomatosis is frequently seen in clinically asymptomatic normal women. Visualization of papillomatosis and parakeratotic changes may be facilitated by acetowhitening — the application of a 3–5% acetic acid solution to the epithelium for 1–2 min. Papillomatosis and acetowhitening in the vulval vestibule are both non-specific findings of uncertain significance and caution is necessary in interpreting the diagnostic significance of epithelium exhibiting these changes.

In cases of symptomatic vestibular papillomatosis, the Committee recommends expert colposcopic examination and the use of acetowhitening primarily as a means of directing biopsies, the results of which should form the basis for therapeutic decisions. Other subgroups have not as yet been officially defined, as diagnostic criteria are not sufficiently established. One such group comprises patients with occasional freedom from symptoms who may have 'cyclic vulvitis', where there is erythema and a sensation of swelling in the acute phase. Another is of patients with no obvious signs on examination but whose symptoms are constant; the term used to describe this group is 'essential vulvodynia'[†]. These women may have some abnormality of cutaneous perception and they often respond to tricyclic antidepressants. Finally, some patients have less easily classified symptoms and do not respond to antidepressants; this group has provisionally been termed idiopathic vulvodynia.

REFERENCE

McKay, M., Frankman, O., Horowitz, B.J. et al. (1991) Vulvar Vestibulitis and Vestibular Papillomatosis: Report of the ISSVD Committee on Vulvodynia. J. Reproductive Med., 36, 413–5.

*Abstracted from McKay et al. (1991).

[†]In discussions of the Committee 1991, it has been proposed that the essential vulvodynia group would be better described as 'dysaesthetic vulvodynia'.

Further reading

Holmes, K.K., Märdh P.-A., Sparling P.F. and Wiesner, P.G. (eds) (1990) *Sexually Transmitted Diseases*, 2nd edition. McGraw Hill, New York.

Ridley, C.M. (ed.) (1988) *The Vulva*. Churchill Livingstone, Edinburgh.

Rook, A., Wilkinson, D.S., Ebling, F.J., Champion, R.H. and Burton, J.L. (eds) (1992) *Textbook of Dermatology*, 5th edition, Blackwell Scientific Publications, Oxford.

Stokes, E.J. and Ridgway, G.L. (1987) *Clinical Microbiology*, Edward Arnold, London.

Index

References in **bold** are to figure numbers

Abscesses 16, 17, **2.19**
Acanthosis nigricans 38, **3.16**
Acrodermatitis enteropathica 88, **6.11**
Acyclovir in genital herpes 25
Adenocarcinoma 71
Adenosquamous carcinoma 71
Adnexal neoplasms 74–5
Alopecia areata 36, **3.12**
Ambiguous genitalia 84, **6.3–5**
Amoebiasis 13, **2.9–11**
Angiokeratoma 66, **4.7–9**
Aphthous ulcers, mouth and vulva 36, **3.9–10**
Apocrine glands 40–1, **3.23, 3.24**

Bartholin's gland and duct abscess 16–17, **2.19–20**
cyst 65, **4.5**
tumours 75
Basal cell carcinoma 38, 72, **3.14, 4.27**
Basal cell papilloma 67, **4.14**
Behçet's syndrome 36, **3.8**
Benzathine penicillin in syphilis 23
11-Beta-hydroxylase deficiency **6.5**
Brugia malayi 11
Bullous dermatoses 41–2
Bullous disease of childhood 88–9, **6.13**
Burning vulva syndrome, *see* Vulvodynia

Calymmatobacterium granulomatosis 20
Candida albicans 14
Candida infection
childhood 91
in diabetes 35, **3.6, 3.35**
Candidosis 14–15, **2.12–15**
Caruncle, urethral 78–9, **5.5**
Cellulitis 71
Cervicitis in genital herpes 24, **2.43**
Cervix
in HPV infection 26

in HSV infection 24, **2.43**
prolapse 80, **5.8**
Trichomonas vaginalis (strawberry) 12, **2.6**
Chancroid 18, **2.24–7**
Childhood tumours, *see* Tumours
Child sexual abuse 95–9, **7.1–6**
investigations for infection 98
Chlamydia trachomatis 23, 98
Cicatricial pemphigoid 43–4, **3.29–33**
Circumcision 82, **5.13**
Clotrimazole
for *Candida* 15
for tinea 15
Colchicine for vulval ulcers 36
Colposcopy 6, **1.2**
acetic acid **1.5**
in HPV infections **2.56–9**
toluidine blue **1.3, 1.4**
Condylomata acuminata, *see* HPV infections
Condylomata lata, *see* Syphilis
Congenital adrenal hyperplasia **6.5**
Corticosteroids, topical
in contact dermatitis 47, **3.42**
in lichen planus 51
in lichen sclerosus, *see* Lichen sclerosus
for lichen sclerosus in childhood 90
in pruritus 49
for vulval ulcers 36
Corynebacterium minutissimum 18, **2.23**
Crohn's disease 34–5, 78, **3.2–4, 5.2**
Cyclosporin, in lichen planus 51
Cystocele 80, **5.7**
Cysts
Bartholin's 65, **4.5**
epidermoid/sebaceous **4.4a,b**
of mesonephric origin **4.2**
mucinous **4.3**

Darier's disease 36
Dermatitis medicamentosa **3.42**
Diabetes 14, 35, **3.6, 3.35**

Diethyl-carbamazine in filariasis 11
Donovanosis 20–1, **2.28–30**

Ectopic tissue 64, **4.1**
Eczema 46, **3.38–40**
Elephantiasis 23, **2.39**
Endometriosis 64, **4.1**
Engorgement
venous, peri-anal, in child sexual abuse 97, **7.6–7**
vulva, neonate 84, **6.5**
Entamoeba histolytica 13
Epidermophyton floccosum 15
Episiotomy, haematoma following 82, **5.12**
Epithelial tumours 67–75
benign 67, **4.12–14**
malignant 71, **4.23–5**
see also Vulval intraepithelial neoplasia
Erysipelas 16
Erythema multiforme **3.25**
Erythrasma 18
in diabetes 35, **3.5**
Erythromycin
for chancroid 18
for erythrasma 18
Escherichia coli, causing Bartholin's abscess 16, 17
Esthiomène 23, **2.39**

Fibro-epithelial polyp 67, **4.12**
Fibromas 64, **4.6**
Filariasis 11
Fissures, anal, in child sexual abuse 97
Fistula, vulval 16, **2.20**
Folliculitis 16, 17, 36, **2.18**
Fox-Fordyce disease 40, **3.23**
Furunculosis, vulval 16–17

Gardnerella vaginalis and child sexual abuse 99, **7.12**
Genetic disorders 36
Genital herpes, *see* Herpes simplex virus infections
Glucagonoma syndrome, vulval manifestations 34, **3.1**

Gonorrhoea 17, **2.21–2**
  Bartholin's abscess 16
  cervical culture 8
  cultures in child sexual abuse 98
  periurethral abscess 17, **2.22**
Granular cell tumour 67, **4.11**
Granuloma inguinale 20–1, **2.28–30**
Griseofulvin for tinea 15

Haemangioma 66, 92, **6.21**
Haematoma following episiotomy 82, **5.12**
Haemophilus ducreyi 18
Haemosiderin 39, **3.18**
Hailey-Hailey disease 36, 44, **3.34**
Hair disorders 36
Hart's line 6, **1.1**
Herpes simplex virus (HSV) infections 24–5, **2.40–7**
  of cervix 24, **2.43**
  in child sexual abuse 98
  in pregnancy 25, **2.45**
Herpes zoster 26, **2.48–51**
Hidradenitis suppurativa 41, **3.24**
Histiocytosis X, *see* Langerhans cell histiocytosis
Human papilloma virus (HPV) infections
  anogenital warts 29–30
  cervix 26
  in children 29–30
  in child sexual abuse 99, **7.9–11**
  Condylomata acuminata 27, **2.53, 2.54, 2.59–61, 2.63**
  giant condyloma 28
  in pregnancy 28, **2.59**
  subclinical 28, **2.56–7**
Hymen, imperforate 84, **6.6**
Hymenal orifice
  in normal child 96, **7.2**
  in sexually abused child 96, **7.2**
Hymenal remnants **4.13**

Imidazoles
  for candidosis 15
  for tinea infection 15
Immunosuppression
  in candidosis 14
  in herpes zoster 26
  in HPV 28
  in HSV 24
  Molluscum contagiosum 31
Inflammatory bowel disease 34–6, 78, **5.2**

Inguinal lymphadenopathy
  in chancroid 18
  in lymphogranuloma venereum 23
  in tuberculosis 11, **2.4**
Intertrigo, vulval 45, **3.35**
Intraepithelial neoplasia, *see* Vulval intraepithelial neoplasia (VIN)

Koebner phenomenon **3.37**

Labial adhesions 84, **6.2**
Langerhans cell histiocytosis 88, **6.12**
Lentigo 38, 72, **4.29**
Letterer-Siwe disease, *see* Langerhans cell histiocytosis
Lichen planus 49–51, **3.47–51**
  erosive 51, **3.49b, 3.53–4**
Lichen sclerosus 52–8
  and child sexual abuse 99, **7.12**
  childhood 90, **6.15–16**
  and squamous cell carcinoma **3.74, 3.75, 4.24, 4.25a,b**
Lichen simplex 48, **3.44–6**
Lichenification
  in eczema 46, **3.38–40**
  in lichen sclerosus **3.68–9**
Linear IgA disease 89, **6.13**
Lymphangioma 67, **4.10**
Lymphoedema
  primary 78, **5.1**
  secondary **5.2, 5.3**
Lymphogranuloma venereum 23, **2.38–9**
Lymphoma, vulval 67

Malathion lotion for pediculosis pubis 11
Melanin-related lesions 38
Melanocytic lesions 72–4, **4.27–31**
  benign 72
  malignant 74
Melanoma 38
  malignant 74, **4.31–3**
Melanosis 38, 72, **4.30**
Metastatic tumours 75
Metronidazole in *Trichomonas vaginalis* 12
Mole 38, 72, 92, **4.28, 6.22**
Molluscum contagiosum 31, **2.65–8**
  childhood 91, **6.19–20**

Nails, lichen planus **3.50**
Napkin rash 86, **6.7–9**
  psoriasiform 87, **6.10**
  seborrhoeic 86–7, **6.9**
Neisseria gonorrhoeae 16, 17, **2.21–2**
Neoplasia
  in childhood 92, **6.21–2**
  epithelial tumours 67
  intraepithelial, *see* VIN
  non-epithelial tumours 65
Normal vulva 6–8, **1.1–6**
Nystatin for candidosis 15

Ovarian carcinoma, metastasis to vulva 75, **4.35**
Oxytetracycline in lymphogranuloma venereum 23

Paget's disease, extramammary **4.21–2**, 70
Papillomatosis
  vestibular 7, 59, **1.5, 3.76**
  classification 104
Patch tests 47, **3.43**
Pediculosis pubis 10, **2.3**
Pemphigoid, cicatricial 43–4, **3.29–33**
Pemphigus, familial benign chronic 44, **3.34**
Pemphigus vulgaris 42–3, **3.27, 3.28**
Penicillin in syphilis 23
Phthirus pubis 10, **2.1, 2.2**
Pigmentation disorders 38–9
Pilonidal sinuses 36
Polyp, fibro-epithelial 67, **4.12**
Post-inflammatory pigmentation 38, **3.15**
Praziquantel in schistosomiasis 11
Procaine penicillin in syphilis 23
Prolapse
  cervix 80, **5.8**
  rectocele 80, **5.9**
  urethral 79, **5.6**
Pseudo-acanthosis nigricans 38, **3.17**
Psoriasiform napkin rash 87, **6.10**
Psoriasis 45, 89, **3.36–7, 6.14**
Punch biopsy 7–8
Pyoderma gangrenosum 35–6, **3.7**
Pyogenic infections 16–17

Radio-necrosis (radiation necrosis) 81, **5.10**

Radiodermatitis 81, **5.11**

Sarcoma 67
Schistosoma haematobium 11
Schistosoma japonicum 11
Schistosoma mansoni 11
Schistosomiasis 11, **2.5**
Sebaceous glands, lesions 40, **3.22**
Seborrhoeic dermatitis 47, **3.41**
Seborrhoeic napkin rash 86–7, **6.9**
Seborrhoeic wart 67, **4.14**
Sexually transmitted diseases,
    investigations 8
    in child sexual abuse 98
Skin tags 67, **4.12**
Squamous cell carcinoma 71, **4.23–5**
    arising on lichen sclerosus **3.74**,
        3.75, **4.24**, **4.25**
Staphylococcus aureus 16, 17
Stevens-Johnson syndrome 41–2,
    3.25
Streptococcal vulvitis
    in child sexual abuse 98, **7.8**
    childhood 91, **6.20**
Streptococcus faecalis, causing
    Bartholin's abscess 16, 17
Streptococcus pyogenes, causing
    erysipelas 16
Sulphamethoxazole for chancroid
    18
Syphilis 21–3, **2.31–6**
    acquired 21
    chancre 21–2, **2.31–3**, **2.36**
    child sexual abuse 98
    congenital 22
    Jarisch-Herxheimer reaction 23,
        2.36

late 22
    secondary 21–2, **2.34–5**
    serological tests 8
Syringomas 74, **4.34**
Systemic diseases, vulval
    manifestations 34–6

Tetracycline hydrochloride
    in granuloma inguinale 21
    in lymphogranuloma venereum
        23
    in syphilis 23
Thrush, *see* Candidosis
Tinea cruris 15, **2.16–17**
Toxic epidermal necrolysis 41–2
Traumatic lesions 82, **5.12–13**
    childhood 92
Treponema pallidum 21–3
Triamcinolone with tetracycline
    for vulval ulcers 36
Trichomonas vaginalis 8, 12, **2.6–8**
Trichophyton rubrum 15
Trimethoprim for chancroid 18
Tumours
    benign, in a child 92
    in childhood 92, **6.21**, **6.22**
    epithelial 67
    malignant, in a child 92, **6.21**
    non-epithelial 65–7

Urethra
    caruncle 78–9, **5.5**
    periurethral abscess 17, **2.22**
    prolapse 79, **5.6**
    tumours 75
Urethritis, acute, in gonorrhoea
    17, **2.21**

Varicosities, vulva 79, **5.4**

Verrucous carcinoma 72, **4.26**
Vestibular papillomatosis 7, 59,
    1.5, **3.76**
    classification 104
Vestibulitis 39, 60–1, **3.18**, **3.77–80**
    classification 104
VIN, *see* Vulval intraepithelial
    neoplasia (VIN)
Viral warts, *see* HPV infections
Vitiligo
    in an adult 39, **3.20–1**
    in a child 91, **6.17**
Vulval intraepithelial neoplasia
    (VIN)
    non-squamous (extramammary
        Paget's disease) 70, **4.21–2**
    squamous 68–9, **4.15–20**
        pigmented 38, **3.13**
        and squamous cell carcinoma
            6, 71, **1.2**, **4.23**
Vulvectomy
    for malignant melanoma 74
    in squamous cell carcinoma 71
    verrucous carcinoma 72
Vulvitis
    streptococcal
        in child sexual abuse 98, **7.8**
        childhood 91, **6.20**
    Zoon's 60
Vulvodynia 59–61, 103–4

Warts, *see* HPV infections
White sponge nevus 36, **3.11**
Wickham's striae **3.48**
Wucheria bancrofti 11

Zinc deficiency **6.11**
Zoon's vulvitis 60